I0820378

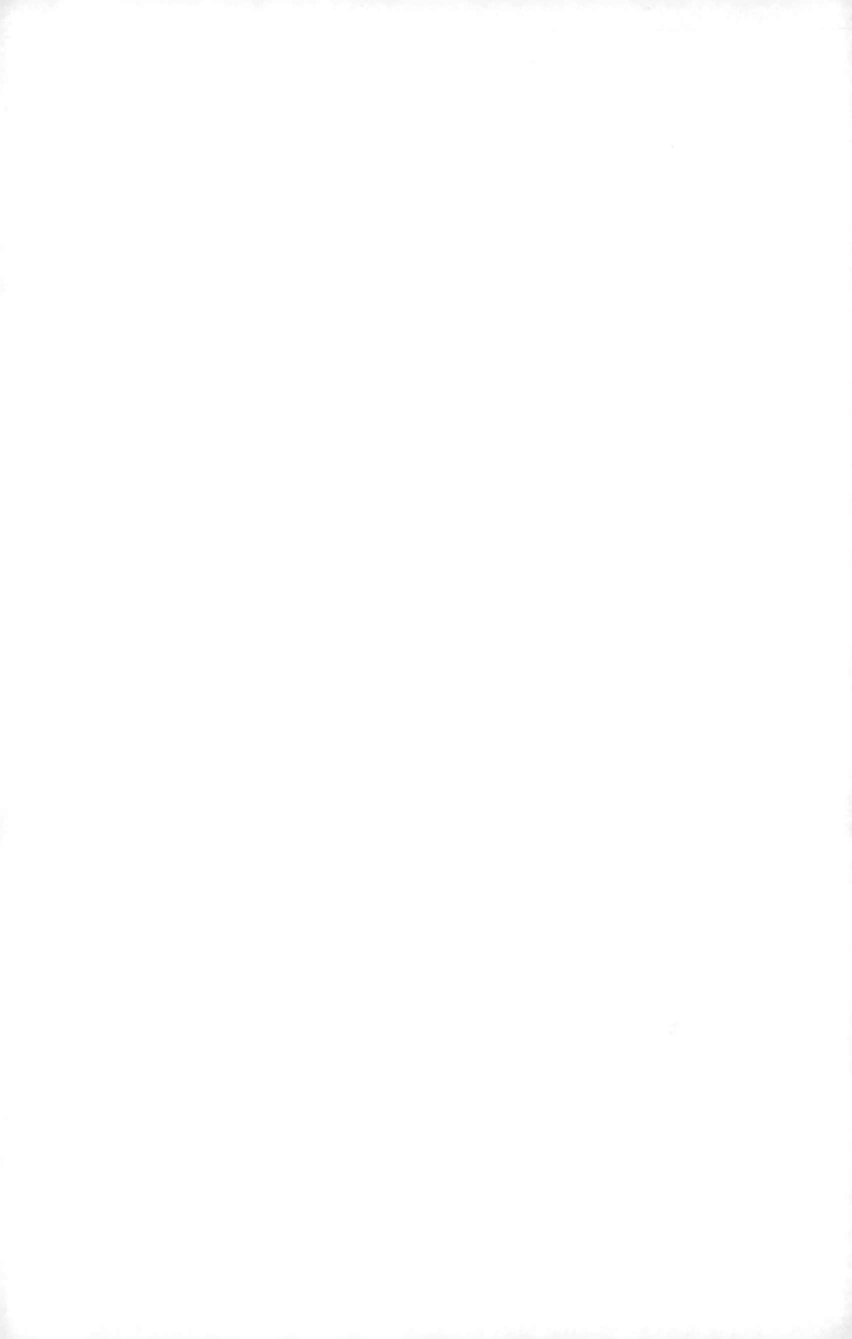

The Art of the *High* Life

The Art of the *High* Life

Unlocking Creativity, Connection, & Relaxation *with* That High Couple

by

Alice and Clark Campbell

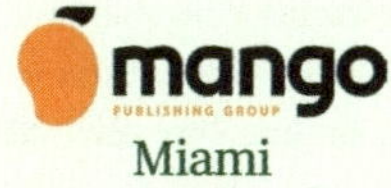

Miami

Published by Mango Publishing, a division of Mango Publishing Group, Inc.

Cover Design, Layout & Design: Megan Werner
Cover Illustration: SERHII / stock.adobe.com
Interior Art Credit: anastasy_helter, artdee2554, Cole, Daria, Dariia, Esgoty, fotohansel, Good Studio, Julia, kolonko, lanastace, marikova, ndog717, North, Sentya Vectors, Visual Generation / stock.adobe.com, Yanka

For permission requests, please contact the publisher at:
Mango Publishing Group
5966 South Dixie Highway, Suite 300
Miami, FL 33143
info@mango.bz

For special orders, quantity sales, course adoptions and corporate sales, please email the publisher at sales@mango.bz. For trade and wholesale sales, please contact Ingram Publisher Services at customer.service@ingramcontent.com or +1.800.509.4887.

The Art of the High Life: Unlocking Creativity, Connection, and Relaxation with That High Couple

Library of Congress Cataloging-in-Publication number: 2024951474

ISBN: (p) 978-1-68481-734-4 (e) 978-1-68481-735-1

BISAC category code: HEA053000 HEALTH & FITNESS / Cannabis & CBD

Contents

Introduction

Hi(gh) friends! We're Alice and Clark, known as That High Couple online, and we're so excited to welcome you into our world of elevated living. For years, we've shared our cannabis adventures on social media, exploring how this plant brings joy, peace, and deeper connection into our lives, enhancing both our relationships and our well-being. Writing *The Art of the High Life* has been a dream; it's a book we hope feels like a friend guiding you through the ways cannabis can enrich your everyday experiences.

Our goal is simple: to help you embrace cannabis as a tool for a more enjoyable and fulfilling life. Whether you're a longtime enthusiast or just starting your journey, we're here to show you how cannabis can be a meaningful part of it. This book isn't just a guide–it's an invitation to explore how cannabis can help you unwind, spark inspiration, and strengthen your connections with the people around you. From choosing your first strain to learning about mindful consumption, we've written *The Art of the High Life* to be both fun and practical.

In the chapters ahead, you'll find thoughtful advice on incorporating cannabis into your daily routine. We'll cover essentials, like navigating a dispensary and finding the right product for different experiences. You'll also discover ideas for enhancing social gatherings, exploring cannabis with your significant other, and even connecting with family. We're diving deep into topics like mental and physical well-being, creativity, and mindfulness while also being conscious of how cannabis fits within the bigger picture of personal wellness.

A huge shout-out to our awesome community—your support and encouragement mean the world to us, and we're so excited to share this book with you. So, here's to new cannabis adventures, stronger relationships, and the art of the high life!

Sending Good Vibes,

Alice & Clark

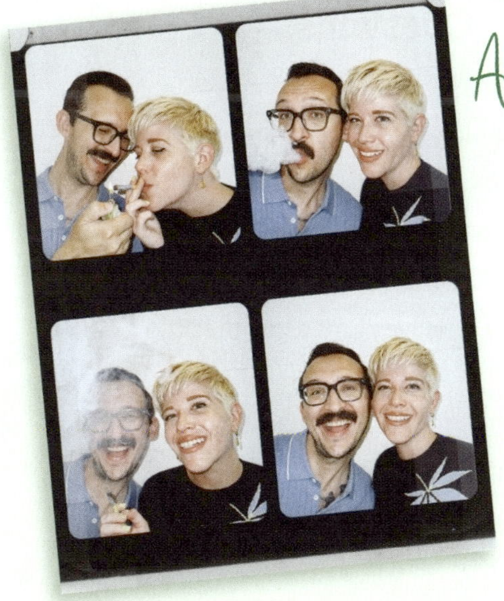

Quiz

What Type of Cannabis Consumer Are You?

Take this quiz to discover your cannabis personality and how to get the most out of this book!

Questions

1. **Why are you most interested in cannabis?**

    A. To manage my stress, sleep better, or feel healthier.

    B. To bond with loved ones and make new memories together.

    C. To spark my creativity and enjoy the little joys of life.

    D. I'm new and curious about how it can enhance my life.

2. **What's your ideal activity to pair with cannabis?**

   A. A calming evening with a cup of tea and a journal.

   B. A laid-back hangout with friends, good vibes, and plenty of laughs.

   C. Painting, writing, or exploring nature.

   D. A cozy movie night while trying an edible for the first time.

3. **How often do you consume cannabis?**

   A. Regularly (daily)—it's part of my wellness routine.

   B. Occasionally (once every few days)—usually in social settings or with my partner.

   C. Sporadically (once every few weeks)—when I want to feel inspired.

   D. Rarely or never (a few times a year)—I'm still figuring out my approach.

4. **What's your favorite way to consume cannabis?**

   A. Tinctures, oils, or topicals—low-key and therapeutic.

   B. Pre-rolls or vapes—easy to share with friends.

   C. Edibles or flower—perfect for enhancing the good vibes.

   D. I don't know yet! I'm excited to explore my options.

5. **When it comes to cannabis, how much do you enjoy learning about it?**

   A. I love diving deep into cannabinoids, terpenes, and wellness benefits.

   B. I like understanding just enough to have a great time with friends.

   C. I enjoy discovering how it connects to creativity and mindfulness.

   D. I'm eager to learn the basics but don't want to get overwhelmed.

6. **What's your ideal cannabis vibe?**

   A. Relaxing and restorative—I'm all about self-care.

   B. Playful and social—I love sharing the experience.

   C. Introspective and creative—I use it to explore new ideas.

   D. Open and experimental—I'm still finding my groove.

7. **What's your biggest concern about using cannabis?**
   A. Overconsumption—I want to make sure I'm using it responsibly.
   B. Social stigma—I worry about what others (friends, family, coworkers, etc.) might think.
   C. Finding the right product—I don't want to waste my time or money.
   D. Everything! I'm a total beginner and need guidance.

8. **How do you feel about cannabis in relationships?**
   A. It's a personal tool for self-care, but I'm open to sharing.
   B. It's a way to deepen connections with friends and family.
   C. It's a shared creative and bonding experience with my partner.
   D. I'm curious about how it could enhance my relationships.

Results

Mostly As: The Wellness-Seeker

You're all about self-care and finding the right balance in life. Whether you're looking for better sleep, stress relief, or a little help with aches and pains, cannabis is your go-to wellness tool. This book will help you dive into cannabinoids, terpenes, and mindful consumption techniques to enhance your physical and mental wellness.

Mostly Bs: The Social Butterfly

For you, cannabis is all about connection and good vibes. You're probably the type who always keeps a pre-roll handy and has the best playlist for the vibe. For you, cannabis isn't just a product; it's the special ingredient that turns good times into great memories. You'll love the sections about group seshes and what activities to pair with different types of cannabis.

Mostly Cs: The Creative Explorer

You see cannabis as your creativity sidekick—a way to think outside the box, find inspiration, and dive into your favorite projects. Whether you're painting, writing, playing music, or just daydreaming about your next big idea, cannabis helps you unlock a deeper sense of flow. You'll find plenty of creative ideas for creative seshes and elevating your imagination.

Mostly Ds: The Curious Newbie

Welcome to the wonderful world of cannabis! The book is your perfect starting point for exploring products, building confidence, and discovering how cannabis can enrich your life. Take it slow and enjoy the journey.

Two As, Bs, Cs, and Ds: An Even Mix

Like with most parts of life, it's hard to pinpoint exactly where we fit in. And that's fine. Rarely is anything in life black and white. You see cannabis as a mixed bag of great experiences, deep thoughts, creative explosions, and self-reflection (good and bad) that sometimes pull you into weed and sometimes push you away. The truth is cannabis can help us untangle our thoughts while also creating new knots. Let's keep that front of mind as we dive into this book!

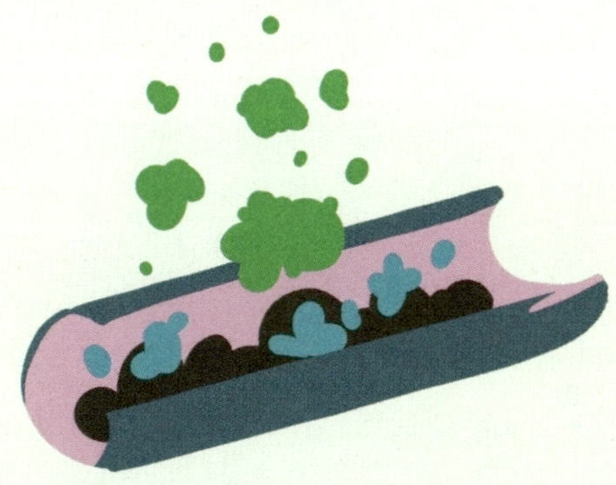

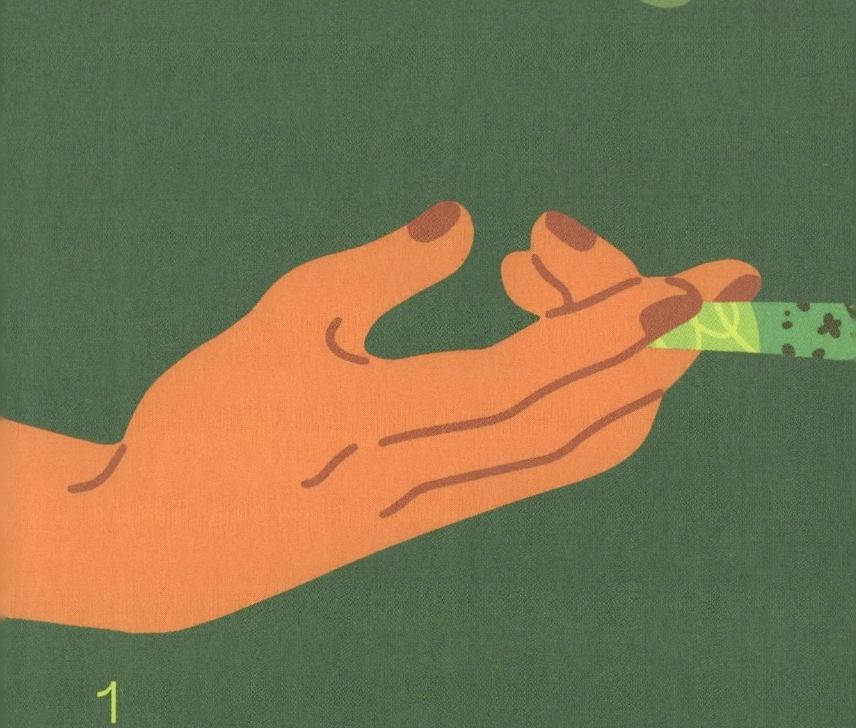

1

Cannabis Basics

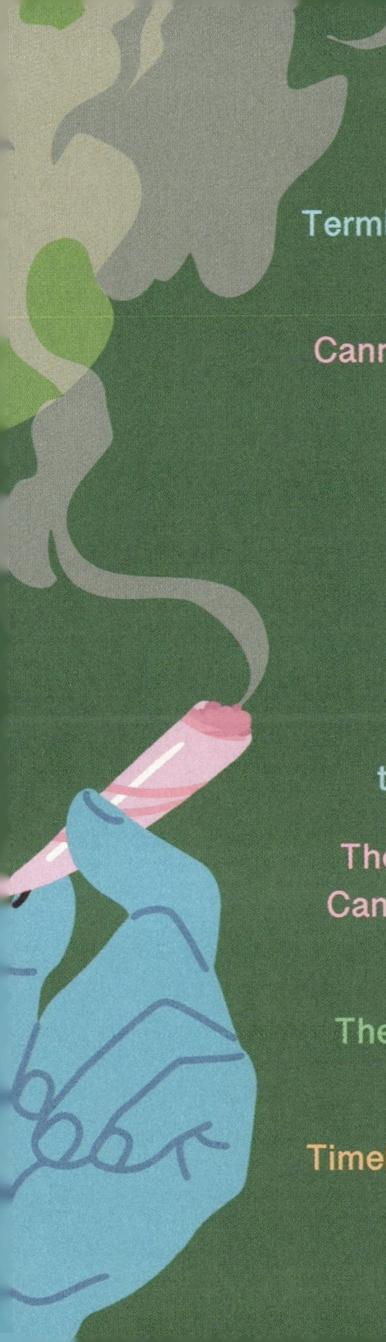

A Glossary of Cannabis Terminology: Key Terms Every Enthusiast Should Know

Cannabis Terms Word Search

Your First Dispensary Visit

How to Converse with a Budtender: Tips & Essential Questions

Finding the Right Places to Enjoy Cannabis Legally

The Ten Commandments of Cannabis Etiquette: Rules for Respectful Consumption

The History of 420: Origins & Cultural Significance

Timeline: The Evolution of 420

A Glossary of Cannabis Terminology

Key Terms Every Enthusiast Should Know

Endocannabinoid System: A network of receptors, molecules, and enzymes found throughout your body. They interact with cannabinoids and can help regulate things like mood, appetite, pain sensation, and memory. It's always good to keep in mind that everyone's endocannabinoid system is different, and that's why the same product might affect different people in different ways.

Strain: A specific variety of cannabis plant. Like how roses or apples offer a lot of different options, think of cannabis the same way. Each strain of cannabis has a unique combination of smell, flavor, and effects. Alice's current favorite stain: MAC (Miracle Alien Cookies). Clark's current favorite strain: Cereal Milk.

Sativa: A type of cannabis plant that's generally known for its energizing and uplifting effects. Alice usually prefers a Sativa!

Indica: Another type of cannabis plant that's generally known for having relaxing and sedative effects. An easy tip for remembering Sativa versus Indica is that an Indica will put you in-da-couch!

Hybrid: A type of cannabis plant that's created by crossing both Sativa and Indica, usually combining qualities from both types. Clark typically gravitates toward hybrid strains, but it's important to note that most strains you encounter aren't strictly Indica or Sativa–they're usually hybrids that feature varying levels of both, along with different levels of cannabinoids. It's all about finding the right balance for the effect you're looking for!

Cannabinoids: These are chemical compounds found in cannabis, including THC and CBD, that interact with your body's endocannabinoid system.

Terpenes: Also called "terps," these are aromatic compounds found in cannabis and other plants that contribute to its flavor, smell, and effects. See Chapter 2 for a breakdown of the most common terpenes found in cannabis.

THC: Tetrahydrocannabinol is the main cannabinoid in cannabis that's responsible for the "high." Fun Fact: THC *also* stands for That High Couple.

CBD: Cannabidiol, a non-intoxicating cannabinoid known for its potential therapeutic benefits, such as relief for pain and anxiety.

Flower: Cannabis has a ton of different nicknames, but we usually see it referred to in a dispensary as "flower" or "bud." This is the actual flowering part of the cannabis plant that contains the highest concentration of terpenes and cannabinoids. It can be smoked in glass like a bong or a pipe, rolled in paper like a joint or a blunt, vaped in a vaporizer, or decarboxylated (heated to around 240 degrees to activate the THC) and used for cooking. Some other nicknames for weed are herb, ganja, Mary Jane, reefer, dank, chronic, devil's lettuce, green, loud, tree, jazz cabbage, and nugs.

Edibles: Cannabis-infused food or beverages. They can range from gummies to mocktails to full-blown infused meals. Edibles take longer to kick in, but the effects will last longer compared to smoking. If you're new to edibles, start with a low dosage (0.5–5mgs), and remember, you can always take more! It's important to note that different kinds of edibles may affect you differently and a lot of the effects can depend on how much you've already eaten that day as well. You can also easily make edibles at home if you have a cannabis vaporizer.

Concentrates: *Highly* potent cannabis extracts made by isolating the plant's cannabinoids and terpenes, often in the form of oils, wax, shatter, diamonds, or hash. If smoking a joint is like drinking a cup of coffee, then taking a dab is like having an espresso. They can be "dabbed," which looks like smoking but involves vaporizing the concentrate versus combusting it like smoking flower. It can also be vaped in a vaporizer made for oils or in a pre-filled vape cartridge.

Topical: A cannabis-infused lotion, cream, or balm that can be applied directly to the skin for localized relief from pain, inflammation, or skin conditions. We both love using CBD lotion on sore muscles after hiking or working out.

Tincture: A liquid cannabis extract often used for sublingual (under the tongue) administration or addition to food and beverages.

Sesh: A "smoke sesh" is what we call the act consuming cannabis.

Consumption Devices

Pipe: A handheld smoking device typically made of glass, metal, wood, or ceramic used to smoke cannabis flower. Alice's first consumption device was a glass, color-changing, mushroom-shaped pipe!

Bong/Bubbler: A water pipe used for smoking flower, which cools and filters the smoke through water for a smoother inhale and larger hit. The difference between a bong and a bubbler is bongs are the big boys of the smoking world; they usually have longer necks and larger chambers. Bubblers, on the other hand, are like the compact, on-the-go version. They still have water filtration but in a smaller, more portable package. We're proud to say we shared a couple of bong hits on our first date together!

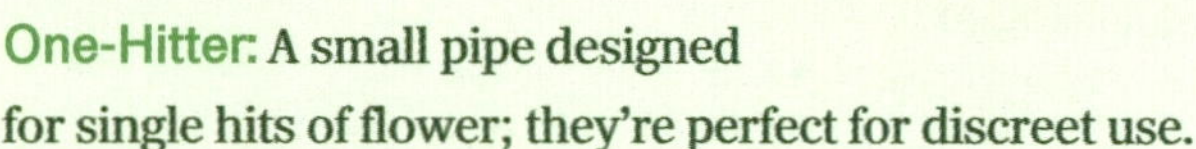

One-Hitter: A small pipe designed for single hits of flower; they're perfect for discreet use.

Joint/Pre-roll: Think of it like a cannabis cigarette made with ground cannabis flower in rolling paper. While we can both roll a smokable joint, it's a skill set we respect! We usually pick up already-rolled joints or "pre-rolls" from the dispensary.

Blunt: Like a joint but rolled in cigar paper or tobacco leaf, often larger and containing more flower.

Spliff: A joint rolled with a combination of cannabis flower and tobacco. These are more popular in the American South and Europe.

Vape: Short for vaporizer, a device used to heat cannabis flower or concentrates to a temperature that releases cannabinoids and terpenes as vapor for inhalation. Vaping is generally more beneficial for your lungs than smoking.

Dab Rig: A water pipe specifically designed for vaporizing cannabis concentrates, usually equipped with a nail or banger for heating the concentrate and requires the use of a hand torch or electronic nail to provide heat. Clark's go-to way to consume at home is with a dab rig after work and a nature documentary on TV.

Cannabis Terms Word Search

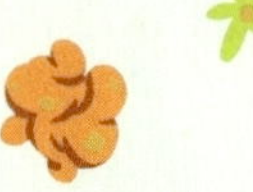

```
A O J M D Z J S B N Z O Z I Z F B U T A K U Y Y Q
T B S V F N V Z G R P Z C E X F U K Y X H B C Y K
V F O T F B V W Z H E P R Q X L B Z T X A H G A E
A P S N O Q L F X I A L U N U O B L Z W J W D I H
P F N C G P E U U F N U Q K I W L S F O Y P M A U
E J C R C F I A N W G D F O T E E E Y S E S H E S
S E N O B O J C H T K W I N Q R R C C Q G G S D X
Y F D S D E J B A K V Z B C V M K H B E W R M I Q
A Z A X M I G A H L F B U J A P E X Y H T W Z B S
D T B M S V F O W D L I L T T Z O W A B U G F L T
D S I N T Y G I N U O B X A E C A W H E R M U E R
F P N N W C B B V T W A A U B Y I Z M V X I H S A
N Z I F C S B I X S E M I F R R R G I D L R D D I
D M I P U T T E F J R Q O A M A I I C B O D O L N
M U S L E F U X D N J O I N T S Z P T V J G Q A T
R M U D P J A R C S S P L I F F A P W J N Q P E H
K M Q E X S X J E U W H V X R X T T O H N H R Y C
L G D R P B K H C B P J C A V Y O V I G Q C I G N
D P G J U I X B H W Q W E B X X H Y V V T D A L M
L S G S D K H Z W W U L M B R R M D K I A Z C M I
```

spliff	topical	flower	vape
strain	indica	hybrid	pipe
flower	sativa	blunt	sesh
bong	thc	cbd	bubbler
tincture	edibles	joint	dab

Your *First* Dispensary Visit

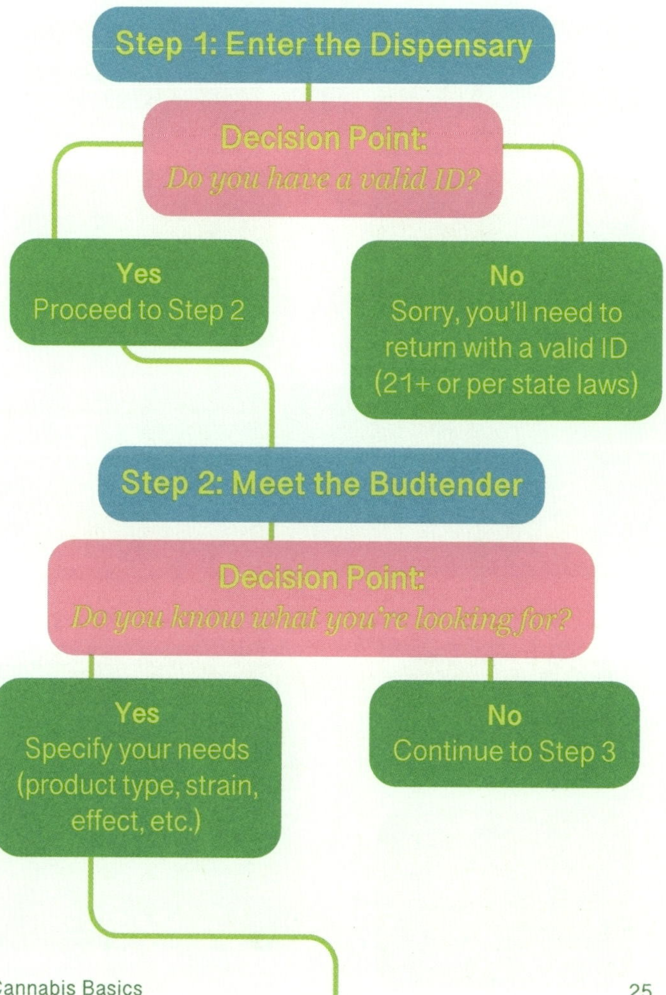

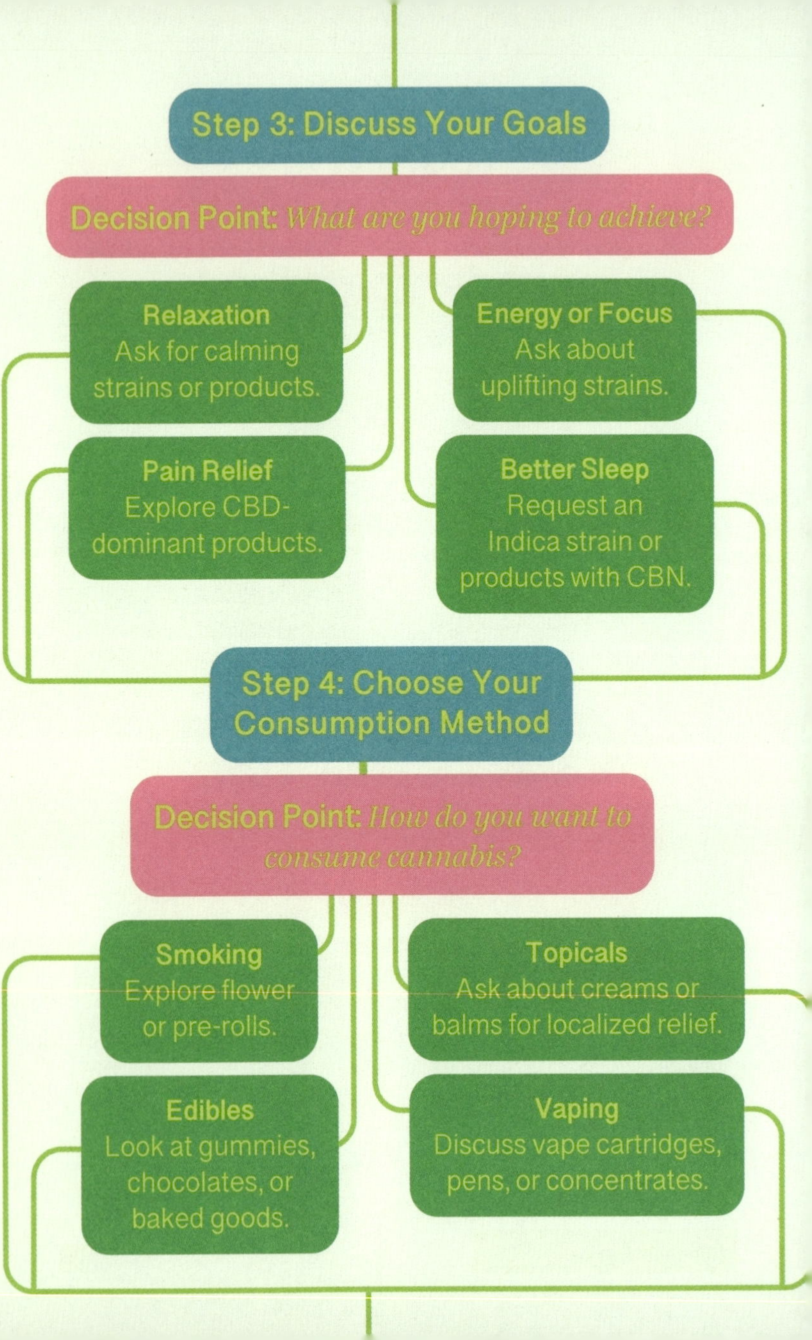

Step 3: Discuss Your Goals

Decision Point: *What are you hoping to achieve?*

Relaxation
Ask for calming strains or products.

Energy or Focus
Ask about uplifting strains.

Pain Relief
Explore CBD-dominant products.

Better Sleep
Request an Indica strain or products with CBN.

Step 4: Choose Your Consumption Method

Decision Point: *How do you want to consume cannabis?*

Smoking
Explore flower or pre-rolls.

Topicals
Ask about creams or balms for localized relief.

Edibles
Look at gummies, chocolates, or baked goods.

Vaping
Discuss vape cartridges, pens, or concentrates.

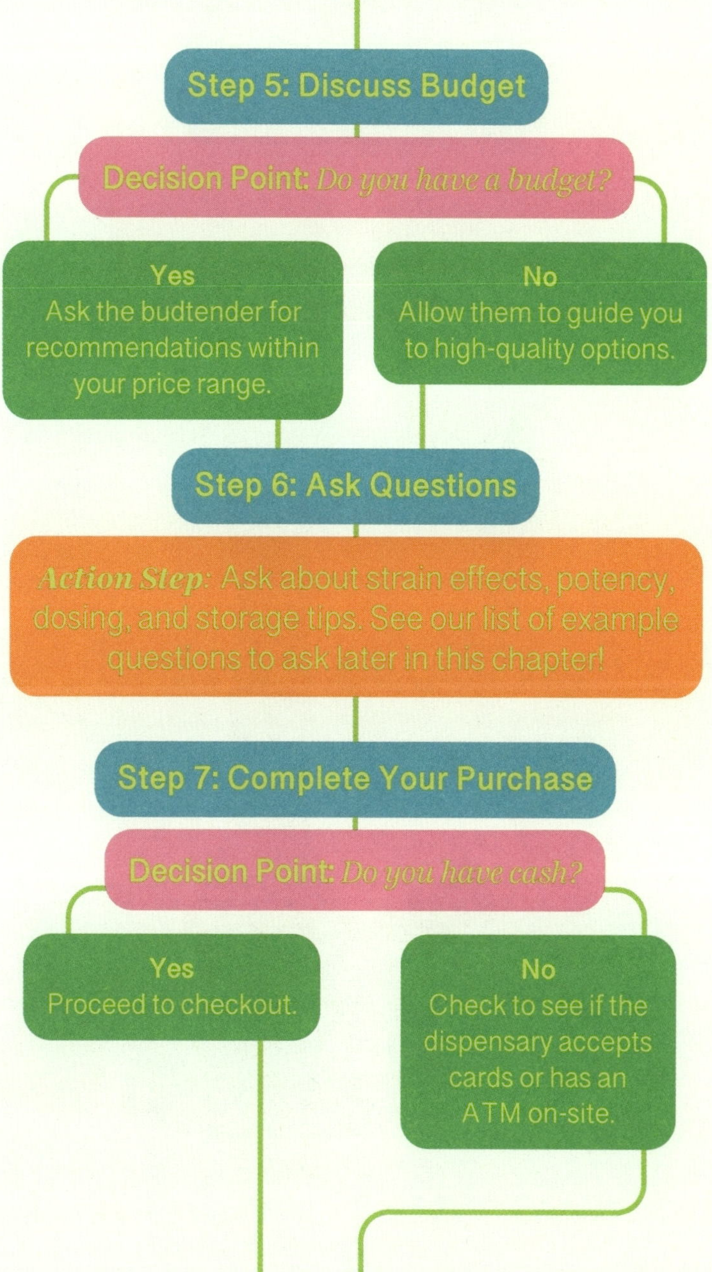

Step 5: Discuss Budget
Decision Point: *Do you have a budget?*
Yes
Ask the budtender for recommendations within your price range.
No
Allow them to guide you to high-quality options.
Step 6: Ask Questions
Action Step: Ask about strain effects, potency, dosing, and storage tips. See our list of example questions to ask later in this chapter!
Step 7: Complete Your Purchase
Decision Point: *Do you have cash?*
Yes
Proceed to checkout.
No
Check to see if the dispensary accepts cards or has an ATM on-site.

Step 8: Enjoy Responsibly

Action Step:
Follow local laws and start with a low dose if you're new.

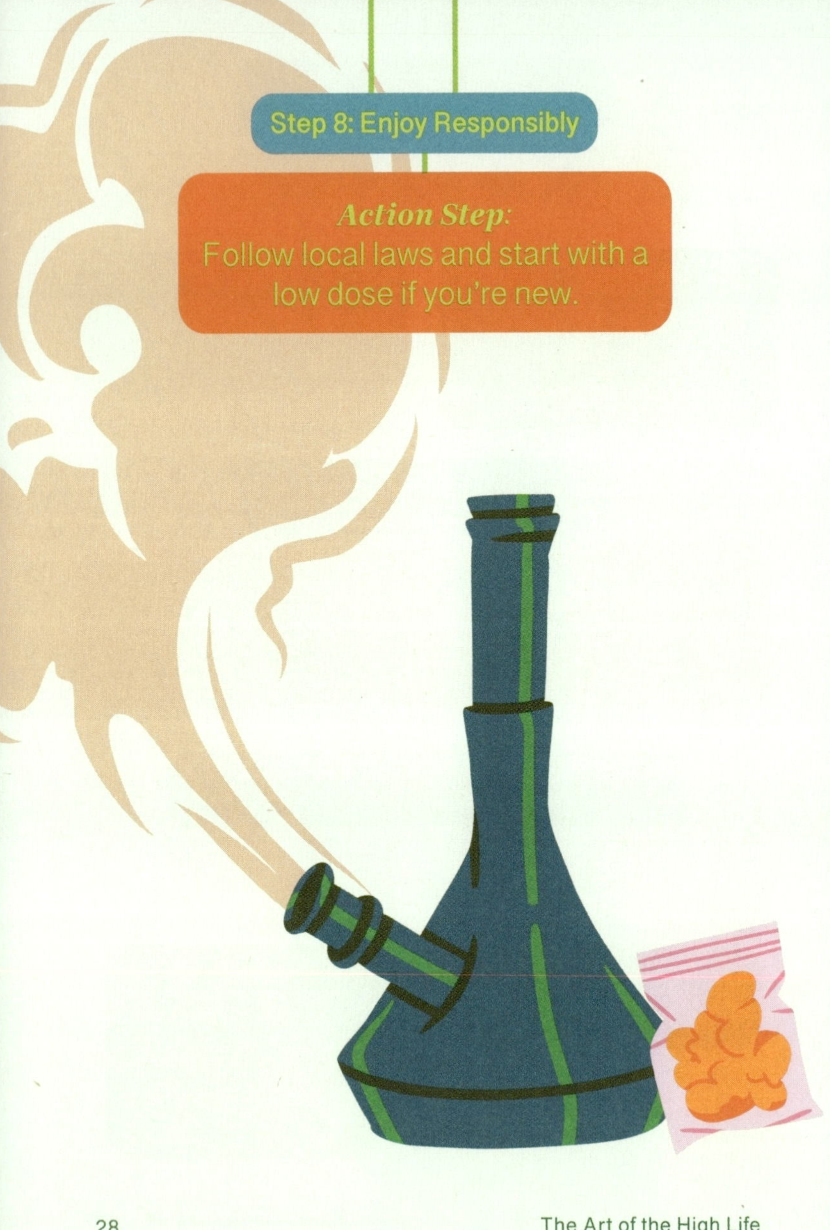

How to Converse with a Budtender

Tips & Essential Questions

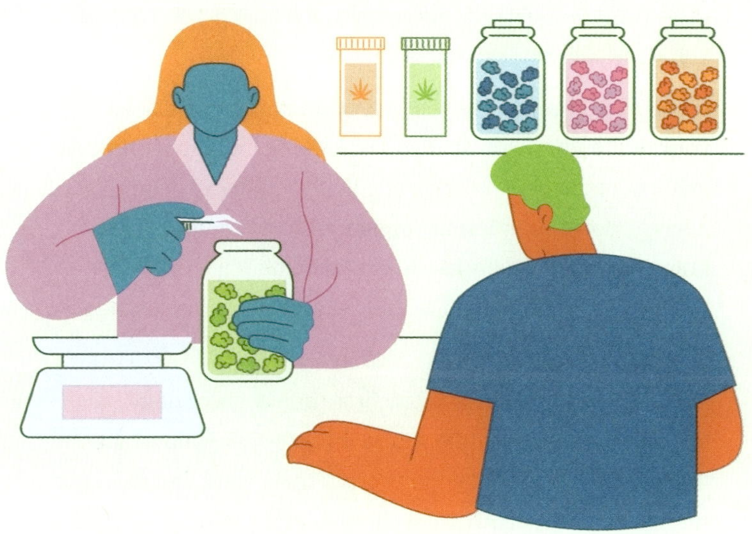

Talking to a budtender can be intimidating if it's your first time. It's important to remember that, like any position, you'll encounter people enthusiastic about their job and others who are just there for the paycheck. That's why it's good to try to be prepared before walking in. Alice has been shopping at dispensaries since she got her first medical marijuana card at age eighteen and Clark spent a year and a half working as a budtender in Hollywood so we feel like we've had plenty of experience on both sides of the counter.

If you don't know where to start when it comes to legally buying cannabis, there's an old saying that holds true—*your nose knows*. Ask if you can smell the flowers; not all dispensaries allow this, but usually, if it smells good to you, you'll probably enjoy that strain.

If you need cannabis to help with something specific, let your budtender know that you're looking for help with sleep, anxiety, motivation, energy, etc. Your budtender should offer a few options for different consumption methods. Let them know how you usually like to consume or, if it's your first time, what you think you're most drawn to (gummies, a preroll, vape cartridge, etc.).

Be sure to ask if they have any first-time deals or daily specials happening while you're there too! We know that "tipping" is somewhat controversial these days, but we think there's no harm in throwing some cash in the tip jar if your budtender helped you choose something you wouldn't have picked out yourself.

Here's a list of questions you can ask your budtender to have a successful shopping experience:

1. What are the **different strains** available, and what are their effects?
2. Can you recommend a strain for (**specific effect or condition**)?
3. What **consumption methods** do you recommend for a beginner?
4. How should I store my cannabis products to **maintain freshness and potency**?
5. Are there any **potential side effects** I should be aware of with certain products or strains?
6. Can you explain the **dosing recommendations**?
7. Are there any **special promotions or deals** available for first-time customers?
8. Are there any **accessories or additional products** you recommend for a beginner?
9. Are there any **legal regulations or guidelines** I should be aware of when consuming the products I've bought here?
10. What are your **personal favorite** products or strains, and why do you recommend them?

Finding the Right Places to Enjoy Cannabis Legally

Some places, like Colorado and California, are lucky enough to have consumption lounges available. This means you can legally buy your cannabis and consume it on-site. If you're in a state without lounges, you're usually restricted to consuming on your own property. Some cities like NYC have public consumption written into their laws so it's always important to read up on what the laws are wherever you'll be consuming. In our time living in Los Angeles, we loved going to the lounges in West Hollywood. One of the most memorable visits was when we went to a tea party at The Studio Cannabis Smoking Lounge located on the second floor of The Artist Tree Dispensary, where we smoked joints, sipped infused tea, and devoured tiny 5mg cakes and sandwiches while they had a violinist playing classic hip-hop covers. Honestly one of our favorite dates!

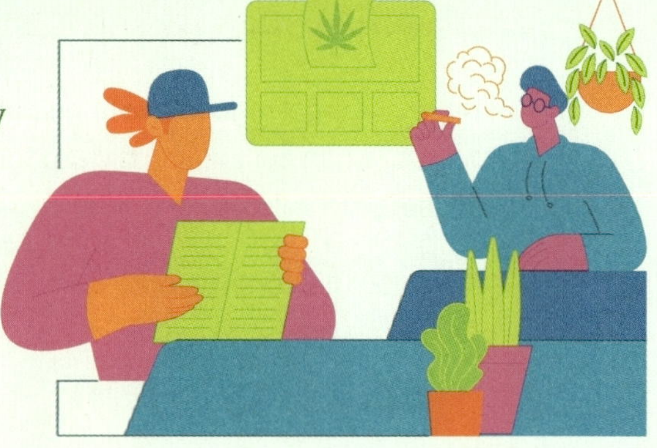

The Ten Commandments of Cannabis Etiquette

Rules for Respectful Consumption

1. **Respect your and others' tolerances**—Everyone's endocannabinoid system is different, along with their tolerance to different kinds of cannabis. Be sure not to push yourself or anyone else you're seshing with to consume more than they should.

2. **Smoke when it benefits you (mindful consumption)**—Try to understand how cannabis can positively impact your well-being by incorporating it into your life in a balanced and responsible way. If you're not already, try to start consuming with intention and an awareness of its effects on your mind and body. A good way to do this is by starting a weed journal. You can keep track of why you're smoking, what you're smoking, and how it makes you feel.

3. **Corner the bowl**—When someone "corners the bowl," they intentionally light only a portion of the flower in the bowl, leaving some unburnt for the next person in the sesh. This preserves the flavor and freshness of the remaining flower, ensuring that everyone gets a green

hit (a hit with fresh, unburnt cannabis) rather than ash or charred remains. Torching a whole bowl that's meant to be shared is kind of like taking a bite out of the middle of a cake rather than cutting it into slices.

4. **Don't steal lighters**—We've all been there...saying goodbye after a sesh and realizing there's a lighter in your pocket that wasn't there before. It's an easy replacement, but try not to be that person!

5. **If you both have flower, make a "salad"**—If you're seshing with a friend and you both have bud, make a salad to be sure you're both contributing to the good vibes.

6. **Don't blow smoke in someone's face (including animals)**—This is self-explanatory, but everyone should be in charge of their consumption. A second-hand high can be uncomfortable for anyone who doesn't sign up for it.

7. **Don't sesh where you shouldn't**—Legally and morally, there are certain places to enjoy cannabis and other places you probably shouldn't. Make sure to check your local laws before consuming and use your common sense. Even if you're in the middle of nature, pay attention to how you're consuming. For example, don't

smoke a joint where lit ashes could potentially hit some dry brush and start a fire.

8. **Never litter**—Another one that's self-explanatory, but dispose of trash in the proper receptacle! It bums us out wherever we see discarded cannabis packaging on the ground. You can take this one step further and plan to sesh before heading out to a local beach or trail to clean up some trash—a great way to enjoy nature and help your community.

9. **Don't "babysit" the bowl/joint**—If you're seshing in a group, be sure to take a hit or two when it's passed to you and then pass it on to the next person. It's understandable, but no one likes it when the person holding the joint spaces out and forgets it's in their hand.

10. **Know what to do if you overconsume**—If you're still figuring out your tolerance level and accidentally overconsume, don't worry; we've compiled some handy tips in Chapter 2 for what to do if you find yourself too high.

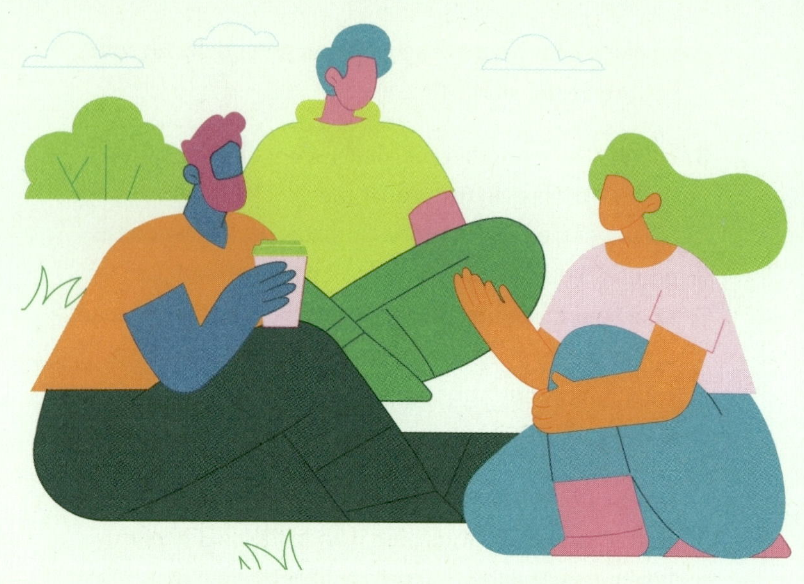

The History of 420

Origins & Cultural Significance

The term "420" has become synonymous with cannabis culture worldwide, and its origins trace back to the early 1970s in San Rafael, California. A group of high school friends, famously known as the "Waldos," began using "420" as a code for meeting up after school to search for a hidden cannabis grow they had heard about. At precisely 4:20 p.m., the Waldos would gather to begin their search and sesh, unknowingly laying the foundation for what would become an iconic symbol in cannabis culture. Their code word remained largely local until they connected with members of the Grateful Dead, a huge part of California music and the hippie scene.

The Grateful Dead, known for their influential role in counterculture, unknowingly helped the term "420" spread as they traveled and shared the code with fans at concerts across the United States. The Waldos' private code became part of the Grateful Dead's wider community, reaching more people with each tour and eventually becoming a common term among cannabis enthusiasts. This quiet spread of "420" was further cemented by *High Times* magazine, which published articles referencing the term and celebrated April 20 as a special day for cannabis. By the early 1990s, "420" was established as a recognized symbol for cannabis culture across the USA and beyond.

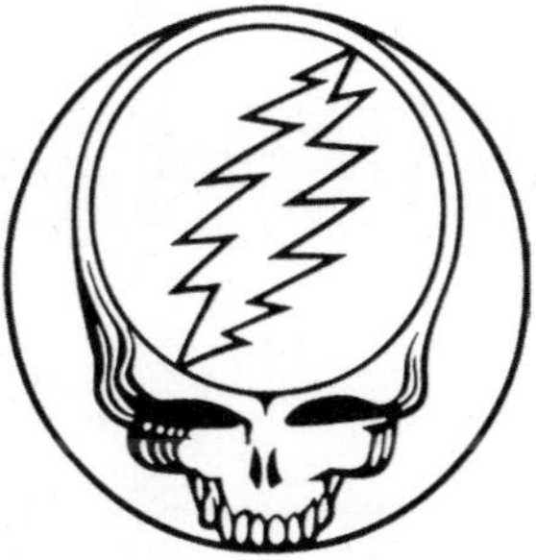

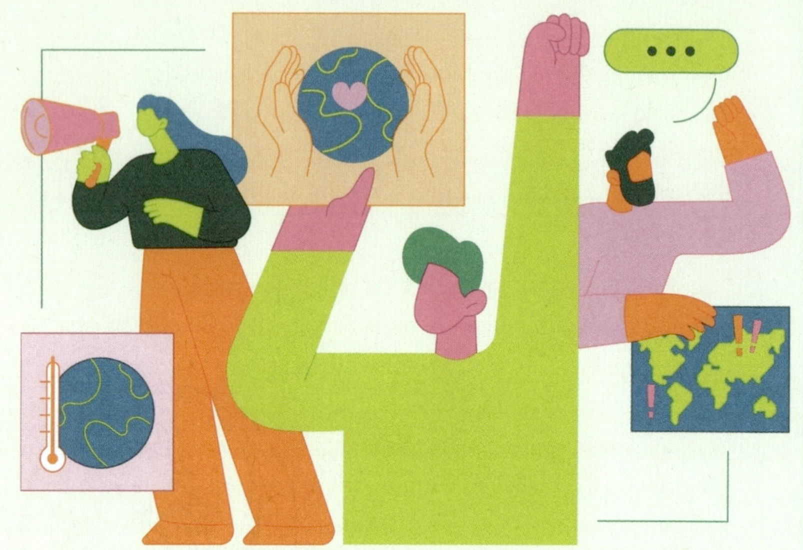

From Code to Celebration

The Cultural Significance of 420

April 20—now celebrated as a global day of cannabis advocacy and community gathering—transcended its original purpose as a meeting code to become something more profound. For many, 4/20 has evolved into a day not just for personal enjoyment but for advocating the normalization and legalization of cannabis. Around the world, cannabis enthusiasts, advocates, and activists come together each

April 20 to participate in festivals, rallies, and protests aimed at spreading awareness and pushing for legal reform.

While the celebratory side of 4/20 is undoubtedly vibrant, with gatherings, concerts, and community events, the day has also become a powerful tool for cannabis advocacy. In countries where cannabis remains illegal or stigmatized, people use April 20 to rally for legalization, engage in public education, and raise awareness about the potential benefits of cannabis for personal well-being and society. For instance, in Canada, where cannabis is fully legalized, April 20 serves as both a celebration of legalization and a reminder of the ongoing advocacy needed in other parts of the world. In Europe and South America, similar gatherings show how the message of 420 extends across cultures and other countries.

The Evolving Meaning of 420

Over the years, 420 has come to mean more than a time or a date–it's become a symbol of acceptance, learning, and good vibes in the cannabis community. Today, 420 stands as a rallying point for those seeking to destigmatize cannabis and break down outdated stereotypes. Many use this day to speak up about responsible consumption, cannabis justice, and equitable access to the industry.

For us, 420 has always been about finding community and advocating for positive change. We began creating cannabis content to share what a mindful, joyful relationship with cannabis looks like and to connect with others who share our vision. Whether you're here to learn, celebrate, or join the conversation, we invite you to embrace 420's deeper significance—both as a day of unity and as a growing movement for a brighter, more inclusive cannabis future.

Timeline

The Evolution of 420

1971: *The Waldos Coin the Code*
A group of high school friends in San Rafael, California, known as "The Waldos," began using "420" as a secret code for meeting up after school to search for a rumored cannabis grow.

1975: *The Grateful Dead Connection*
The Waldos' code spread through their connection to the Grateful Dead, who were central to California's music and counterculture scene. Fans adopted "420" as a symbol of cannabis use.

1990: ***High Times* Amplifies 420**

High Times magazine published references to 420, popularizing the term beyond California. They began promoting April 20 as a day for cannabis enthusiasts to celebrate.

1995: ***April 20 Becomes a Movement***

Cannabis activists began using April 20 as a day of advocacy, pushing for legalization and normalization of cannabis use.

2012: ***Legalization Milestones***

Colorado and Washington became the first US states to legalize recreational cannabis, setting the stage for 420 celebrations to take on new significance.

2018: ***Canada Legalizes Cannabis***

Canada fully legalized cannabis, making 420 a day of celebration and reflection on progress.

Today: ***A Global Cannabis Holiday***

April 20 is celebrated worldwide as a day for cannabis advocacy, community gatherings, and education about responsible consumption.

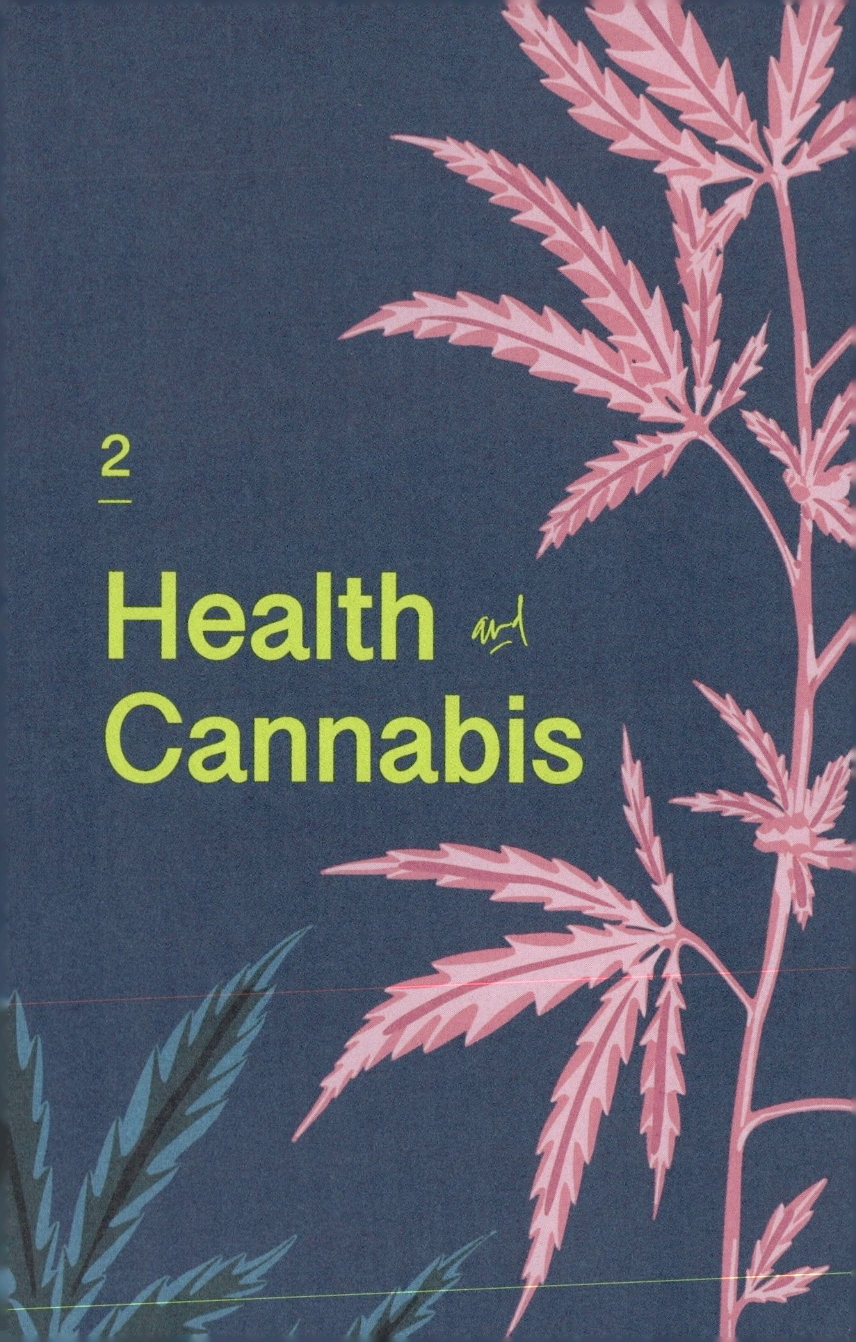

2

Health and Cannabis

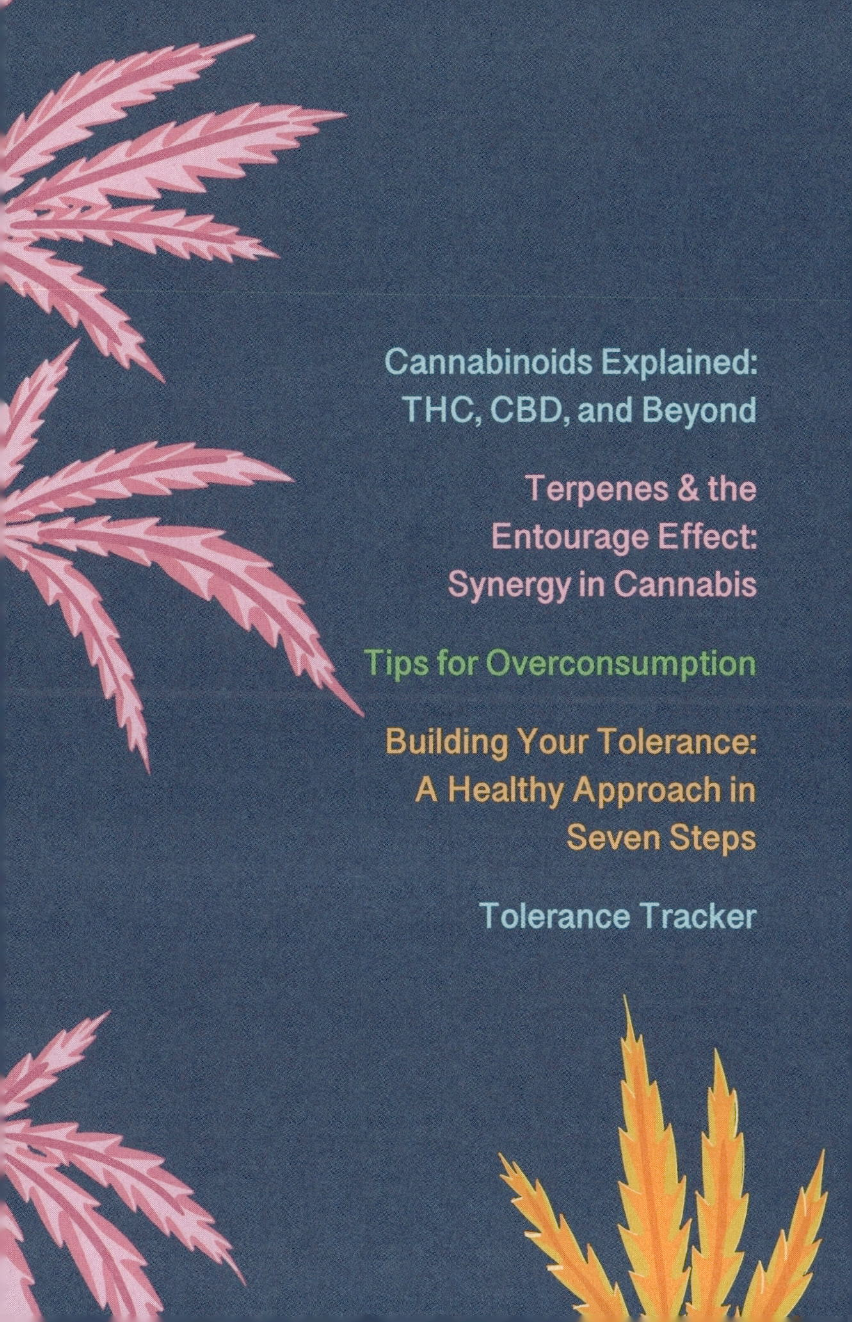
Cannabinoids Explained:
THC, CBD, and Beyond
Terpenes & the
Entourage Effect:
Synergy in Cannabis
Tips for Overconsumption
Building Your Tolerance:
A Healthy Approach in
Seven Steps
Tolerance Tracker

Cannabinoids Explained
THC, CBD, and Beyond

The two main cannabinoids you've probably heard of are THC and CBD. THC is what gets you high and giggly. It's the party starter of the bunch. CBD, on the other hand, is way more chill. It doesn't get you intoxicated, but it does have some amazing potential therapeutic benefits, like helping with pain, anxiety, and inflammation.

But here's the thing—those are just the tip of the iceberg! Over one hundred different cannabinoids are in the cannabis plant, each with unique effects and potential benefits. There's no need to be versed in *all* of them, but a few main cannabinoids worth looking out for are:

- **CBG (Cannabigerol):** Often referred to as the "mother cannabinoid" because it's the precursor to other cannabinoids like THC and CBD. CBG is non-intoxicating and is being researched for its potential to help with inflammation and other health issues.

- **CBN (Cannabinol):** Cannabinoid is formed when THC ages or when it's exposed to oxygen and light. It's mildly psychoactive but is mostly known for its sedative effects. Some research suggests that CBN may have potential as a sleep aid. It's also often found in aged cannabis and is more than likely contributing to the "couch-lock" sensation that some people experience when smoking older flower. One time, we held onto a bottle of THC-infused non-alcoholic wine for a couple of years before opening it, and when we finally did, we were both asleep on the couch by 9:00 p.m. that night! We're almost positive the THC had turned to CBN in the years it spent sitting on our wine rack—oops!

- **THCV (Tetrahydrocannabivarin):** Like THC but with a slightly different molecular structure, THCV is known for its potential appetite-suppressing and energizing effects. We ran our first 5k race in Los Angeles with the help of some THCV gummies we enjoyed before and after the run!

- **CBC (Cannabichromene):** While not as well-known as THC or CBD, CBC is gaining attention for its potential anti-inflammatory and antidepressant properties. It doesn't produce intoxicating effects on its own but may enhance the effects of other cannabinoids.

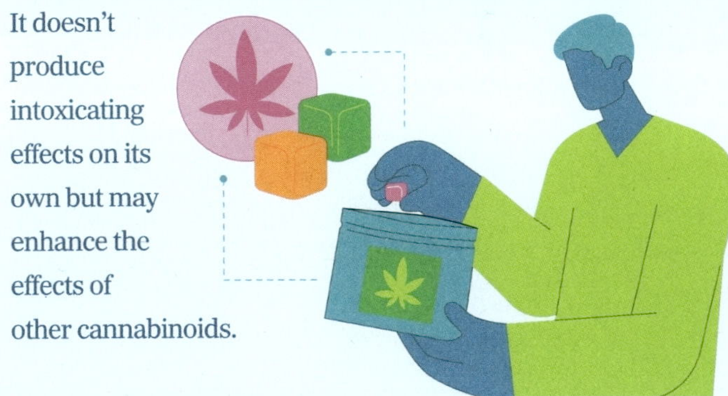

Terpenes & the Entourage Effect

Synergy in Cannabis

Let's talk terps! Terpenes are more common than you may think and are found in a variety of other plants and foods besides cannabis. They're responsible for the unique smells and flavors of different strains. But there's an even deeper layer to it–terpenes also interact with cannabinoids in a phenomenon known as the entourage effect. **cue the angelic choir**

The entourage effect is all about synergy, baby! It's the idea that cannabinoids and terpenes work together to enhance each other's effects. For example, certain terpenes might help cannabinoids like THC or CBD enter your bloodstream more efficiently, potentially making their effects stronger and longer lasting.

But it's not just about potency. Terpenes also contribute to the overall experience of consuming cannabis. Have you ever smelled a strain and immediately felt relaxed or uplifted? Those are the terpenes at work! They have the power to influence your mood, energy, and stress levels–think "aromatherapy."

So, when it comes to choosing a strain, it's not just about Sativa or Indica or even how high the THC or CBD percentage is. It's important to pay attention to the terpenes as well! Whether you're looking for something calming, energizing, or somewhere in between, the right combination of cannabinoids and terpenes can make all the difference in your experience.

In essence, terpenes and cannabinoids are like the dynamic duo of cannabis, working together to create a symphony of effects that's greater than the sum of its parts. It's nature's way of giving us a little something extra with every puff!

A few of the most common terpenes to familiarize yourself with are:

- **Myrcene:** Myrcene is one of the most common terpenes in cannabis and is known for its earthy and musky scent. To us, Myrcene always smells like some herb combo that we can't place our finger on. It's often associated with relaxing, chill, and sedative effects. You'll find it in strains like Blue Dream and Granddaddy Purple. But you'll also find Myrcene in things like mangoes, hops, thyme, and lemongrass.

- **Limonene:** Limonene has a bright and citrusy aroma that's easy to identify. It's uplifting and can help with mood elevation and stress relief. You can find limonene in cannabis strains like Super-

Lemon Haze and Dosidos. But you can also find it in lemons, oranges, limes, and juniper.

- **Pinene:** Pinene smells like—you guessed it—pine! It's refreshing and can help with alertness and memory retention. You'll find pinene in strains like Cherry Bomb and Crunch Berries and in things like pine needles (duh), rosemary, basil, and parsley.

- **Linalool:** Linalool has a floral, lavender-like aroma. It's known for its calming, anti-anxiety, and antidepressant properties. Linalool is the main terpene in the strains Durban and Alice's favorite, MAC. It's also present in lavender, coriander, birch bark, and rosewood.

- **Caryophyllene:** Caryophyllene, also sometimes called Beta-Caryophyllene, has a spicy, peppery scent. It's believed to have potentially anti-inflammatory benefits. You'll find it in strains like Girl Scout Cookies (GSC), Bubba Kush, and Clark's favorite, Cereal Milk. You'll also find it in things like black pepper, cloves, cinnamon, and basil.

- **Terpinolene:** Terpinolene has a complex aroma–floral, herbal, and slightly citrusy. It's known for its uplifting effects and potential antioxidant properties. You'll find terpinolene in strains like Jack Herer as well as in apples, cumin, lilacs, and tea tree oil.

- **Humulene:** Humulene has a woody, earthy smell and is known for its anti-inflammatory and appetite-suppressing effects. It's sometimes found in smaller quantities versus the other terpenes listed above, but you can still note it in strains like Headband and Death Star, along with things like hops, coriander, basil, and clove.

Understanding these terpenes can help you choose the right strain for your desired effects and experience. Plus, it's cool to know that these compounds are found in everyday plants and foods!

Tips for Overconsumption

Please remember that we aren't doctors, and nothing in this book should be taken as medical advice. We're just two cannabis enthusiasts who have found some success with the following suggestions! The first thing to do is not panic;

remember that this is a temporary state, and you're not in any real danger. It's impossible to overdose on cannabis. Estimates say that you'd need to smoke around 1,500 pounds of cannabis in the span of about fifteen minutes to overdose; that's around twenty to forty thousand joints! No one has ever died from cannabis overconsumption in the history of mankind, and you won't be the first.

Next, find a safe environment, somewhere you can get comfy cozy and drink a nice, tall glass of water. Drinking water is a great way to detoxify your body, so try to drink plenty of it.

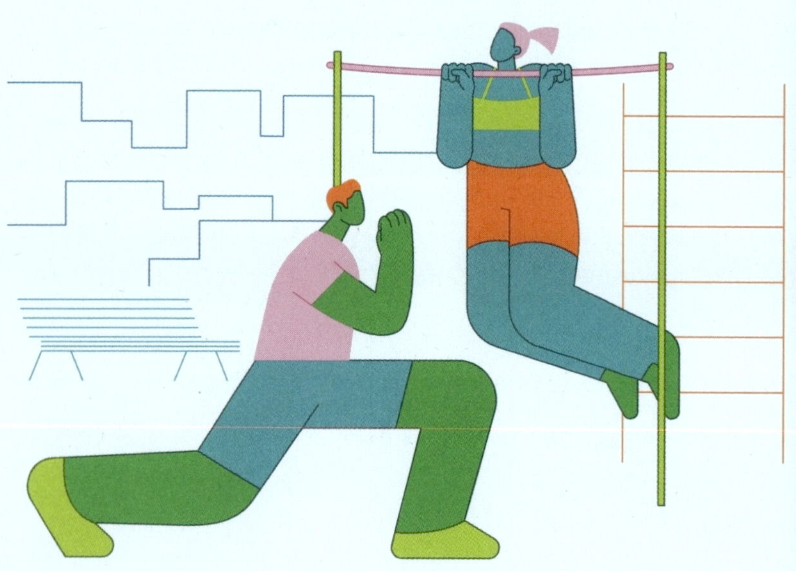

If you're at home and happen to have any fresh lemons or black pepper around, the terpenes limonene and caryophyllene are known to help alter THC's effects in the brain. Squeezc out and take a shot of lemon juice or get a good whiff of some lemon zest or fresh ground pepper. If you're worried about sneezing when smelling the pepper, try chewing on some of the peppercorns or sucking on them under your tongue.

If you're still feeling sluggish after your lemon pepper smoothie, try exercising. It's a great way to sober up in a hurry because it causes a release of endorphins. If you can exercise outside, the fresh air and sunshine aren't bad for you either!

Weed and munchies also go hand in hand for a reason. If you've eaten an edible that you need to dilute a little, get some snacks into that tummy! It's important to remember that different foods can help in different ways. If you're feeling anxious, scatterbrained, or paranoid, try drinking some calming tea or eating foods high in dairy content. Those should help to coat the inside lining of your stomach to help prevent any more THC from getting into your system. If you're feeling too couch-locked or lazy, try drinking a cup of coffee or eating foods high in water content, like grapefruit. You can also try chewing minty gum to help get you stimulated.

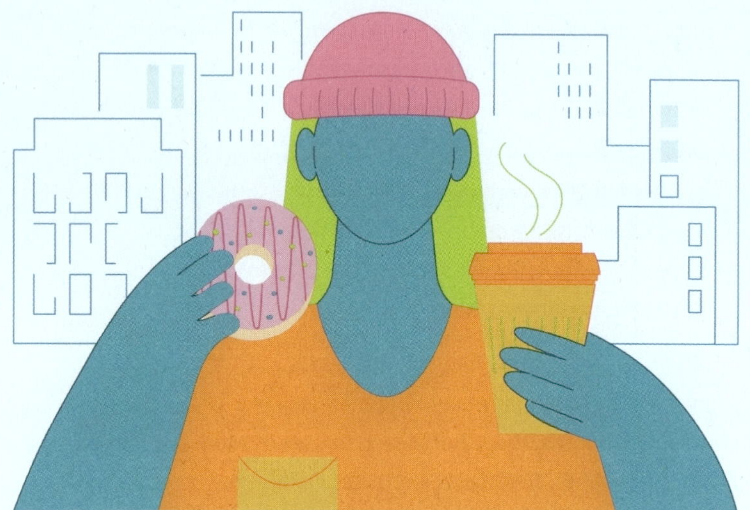

If you feel like you're so high that you're on the verge of "blacking out," go ahead and do it! Close your eyes and take a nice little nap. There shouldn't be any fear of going to sleep while you're high. Keep in mind that depending on how high you are, don't be surprised if you wake up and you're still feeling it. One Friday afternoon, we split a 1,000mg brownie (can't say we recommend it) and woke up on Monday morning still feeling the effects. We didn't get scared though because we knew the feeling was temporary and would eventually pass (it did later that day).

There's one last thing we can recommend to get you off this crazy cannabis roller coaster if you're still feeling stuck. CBD can be great for combating the effects of THC. You can think of it as the yin to THC's yang. It can work to block THC from binding to the cannabinoid receptors in your brain, thus toning down the high effects. The quickest way to get CBD into your system is by taking a few drops of CBD tincture under your tongue, but we almost always have a pure CBD oil vape pen lying around as well to take a few puffs from, just in case.

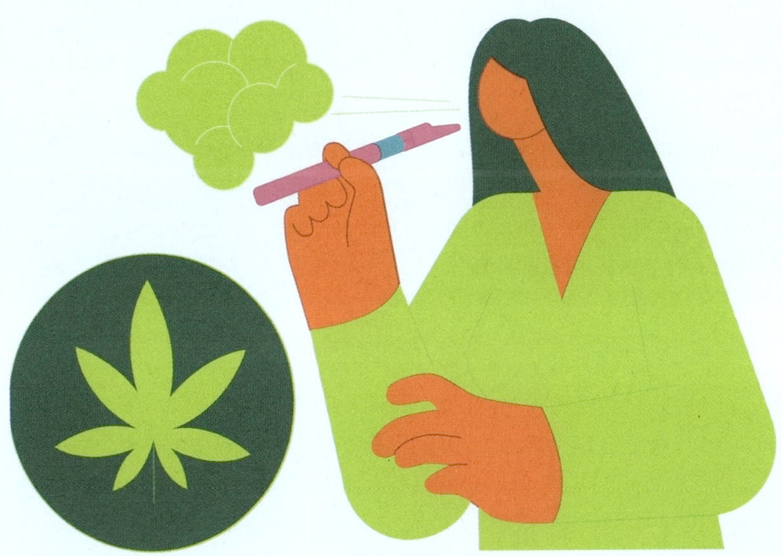

Building Your Tolerance

A Healthy Approach in Seven Steps

There are plenty of reasons why someone would want to build up their tolerance to cannabis. Whether you're new to the scene or looking to manage your consumption better, these seven steps can help you navigate your cannabis journey responsibly.

1. Start Low and Go Slow

When you're new to cannabis or trying a new product, always start with a low dose. This approach helps you understand how your body reacts without overwhelming your system. Remember, you can always take more, but you can't take less once you've consumed.

2. Choose the Right Strain

Different strains have different effects. Some are high in THC, while others are rich in CBD. Start with strains that have balanced or lower THC content to help you build tolerance gradually. Pay attention to the terpenes present in the strains you like and don't like so you know where to go from there. You can also ask your budtender for recommendations.

3. Stay Consistent

Consistency is key when building tolerance. Try to consume similar amounts at regular intervals. This helps your body adapt and prevents sudden spikes in tolerance. As we mentioned in Chapter 1, it can also help to track your consumption with a journal or an app.

4. Hydrate and Eat Well

Staying hydrated and maintaining a balanced diet can make a significant difference in how your body handles cannabis. Water helps flush out toxins, while a good diet supports overall health. We would also recommend avoiding consuming cannabis on an empty stomach.

5. Take Tolerance Breaks

Even seasoned users (like us) benefit from taking breaks. A tolerance break, or "T-break," allows your body to reset and become more sensitive to THC again. Consider taking a few days to a couple of weeks off every few months to maintain a manageable tolerance level. We love to travel, so we usually have a built-in T-break whenever we take an international vacation.

6. Mix Up Your Methods

Try experimenting with different consumption methods like edibles, vapes, tinctures, and topicals. Each method has a different onset time and duration, which can help you understand what works best for you and prevent overconsumption.

7. Listen to Your Body

Your body knows best. Pay attention to how you feel before, during, and after consuming cannabis. If you start feeling uncomfortable or notice negative effects, scale back your usage or take a break. Mindful consumption ensures a positive and enjoyable experience.

Building your cannabis tolerance is a personal journey, and there's no one-size-fits-all approach. By starting low, staying consistent, and listening to your body, you'll find the perfect balance that enhances your life without overwhelming you. Remember to stay lifted and enjoy the ride!

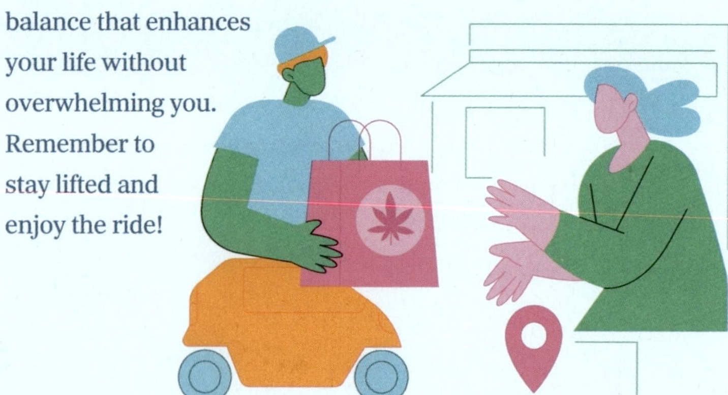

Tolerance Tracker

Date:	Strain/Method Tried:
Dosage:	Mood Before: & After:

Notes on Experience:

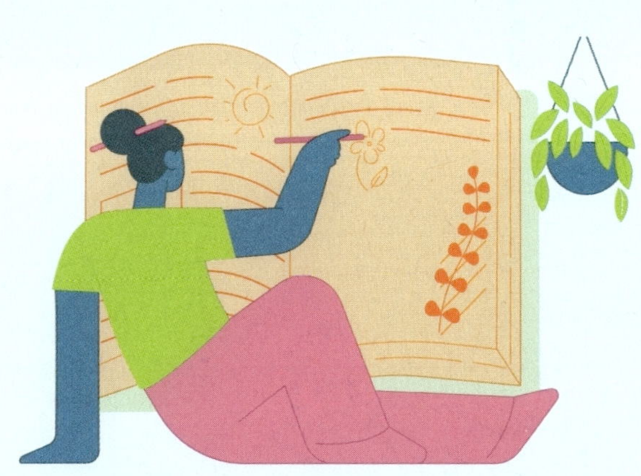

Date:	Strain/Method Tried:
Dosage:	Mood Before: & After:

Notes on Experience:

Date:	Strain/Method Tried:
Dosage:	Mood Before: & After:

Notes on Experience:

Date:	Strain/Method Tried:
Dosage:	Mood Before: & After:

Notes on Experience:

Date:	Strain/Method Tried:
Dosage:	Mood Before: & After:

Notes on Experience:

Date:	Strain/Method Tried:
Dosage:	Mood Before: & After:

Notes on Experience:

Date:	Strain/Method Tried:
Dosage:	Mood Before: & After:

Notes on Experience:

Date:	Strain/Method Tried:
Dosage:	Mood Before: & After:

Notes on Experience:

Date:	Strain/Method Tried:
Dosage:	Mood Before: & After:

Notes on Experience:

Date:	Strain/Method Tried:
Dosage:	Mood Before: & After:

Notes on Experience:

Date:	Strain/Method Tried:
Dosage:	Mood Before: & After:

Notes on Experience:

Date:	Strain/Method Tried:
Dosage:	Mood Before: & After:

Notes on Experience:

Date:	Strain/Method Tried:
Dosage:	Mood Before: & After:

Notes on Experience:

Date:	Strain/Method Tried:
Dosage:	Mood Before: & After:

Notes on Experience:

Date:	Strain/Method Tried:
Dosage:	Mood Before: & After:

Notes on Experience:

Date:	Strain/Method Tried:
Dosage:	Mood Before: & After:

Notes on Experience:

Date:	Strain/Method Tried:
Dosage:	Mood Before: & After:

Notes on Experience:

Date:	Strain/Method Tried:
Dosage:	Mood Before: & After:

Notes on Experience:

Date:	Strain/Method Tried:
Dosage:	Mood Before: & After:

Notes on Experience:

Date:	Strain/Method Tried:
Dosage:	Mood Before: & After:

Notes on Experience:

Date:	Strain/Method Tried:
Dosage:	Mood Before: & After:

Notes on Experience:

Date:	Strain/Method Tried:
Dosage:	Mood Before: & After:

Notes on Experience:

Date:	Strain/Method Tried:
Dosage:	Mood Before: & After:

Notes on Experience:

Date:	Strain/Method Tried:
Dosage:	Mood Before: & After:

Notes on Experience:

____

____

____

____

Date:	Strain/Method Tried:
Dosage:	Mood Before: & After:

Notes on Experience:

____

____

____

____

Date:	Strain/Method Tried:
Dosage:	Mood Before: & After:

Notes on Experience:

____

____

____

____

Date:	Strain/Method Tried:
Dosage:	Mood Before: & After:

Notes on Experience:

____

____

____

____

Date:	Strain/Method Tried:
Dosage:	Mood Before: & After:

Notes on Experience:

Date:	Strain/Method Tried:
Dosage:	Mood Before: & After:

Notes on Experience:

Date:	Strain/Method Tried:
Dosage:	Mood Before: & After:

Notes on Experience:

____

____

____

____

Date:	Strain/Method Tried:
Dosage:	Mood Before: & After:

Notes on Experience:

____

____

____

____

Date:	Strain/Method Tried:
Dosage:	Mood Before: & After:

Notes on Experience:

Date:	Strain/Method Tried:
Dosage:	Mood Before: & After:

Notes on Experience:

Date:	Strain/Method Tried:
Dosage:	Mood Before: & After:

Notes on Experience:

____

____

____

____

Date:	Strain/Method Tried:
Dosage:	Mood Before: & After:

Notes on Experience:

____

____

____

____

Date:	Strain/Method Tried:
Dosage:	Mood Before: & After:

Notes on Experience:

____

____

____

____

Date:	Strain/Method Tried:
Dosage:	Mood Before: & After:

Notes on Experience:

____

____

____

____

Date:	Strain/Method Tried:
Dosage:	Mood Before: & After:

Notes on Experience:

Date:	Strain/Method Tried:
Dosage:	Mood Before: & After:

Notes on Experience:

Date:	Strain/Method Tried:
Dosage:	Mood Before: & After:

Notes on Experience:

Date:	Strain/Method Tried:
Dosage:	Mood Before: & After:

Notes on Experience:

Date:	Strain/Method Tried:
Dosage:	Mood Before: & After:

Notes on Experience:

Date:	Strain/Method Tried:
Dosage:	Mood Before: & After:

Notes on Experience:

Date:	Strain/Method Tried:
Dosage:	Mood Before: & After:

Notes on Experience:

____

____

____

____

Date:	Strain/Method Tried:
Dosage:	Mood Before: & After:

Notes on Experience:

____

____

____

____

Date:	Strain/Method Tried:
Dosage:	Mood Before: & After:

Notes on Experience:

Date:	Strain/Method Tried:
Dosage:	Mood Before: & After:

Notes on Experience:

Date:	Strain/Method Tried:
Dosage:	Mood Before: & After:

Notes on Experience:

Date:	Strain/Method Tried:
Dosage:	Mood Before: & After:

Notes on Experience:

Date:	Strain/Method Tried:
Dosage:	Mood Before: & After:

Notes on Experience:

Date:	Strain/Method Tried:
Dosage:	Mood Before: & After:

Notes on Experience:

Date:	Strain/Method Tried:
Dosage:	Mood Before: & After:

Notes on Experience:

____

____

____

____

Date:	Strain/Method Tried:
Dosage:	Mood Before: & After:

Notes on Experience:

____

____

____

____

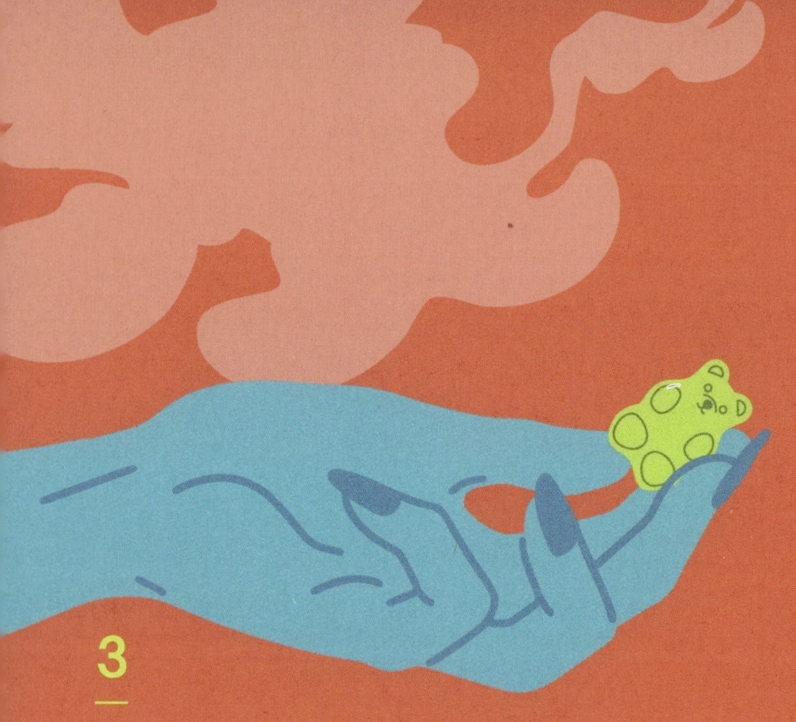

3

Enhancing Happiness *with* Cannabis

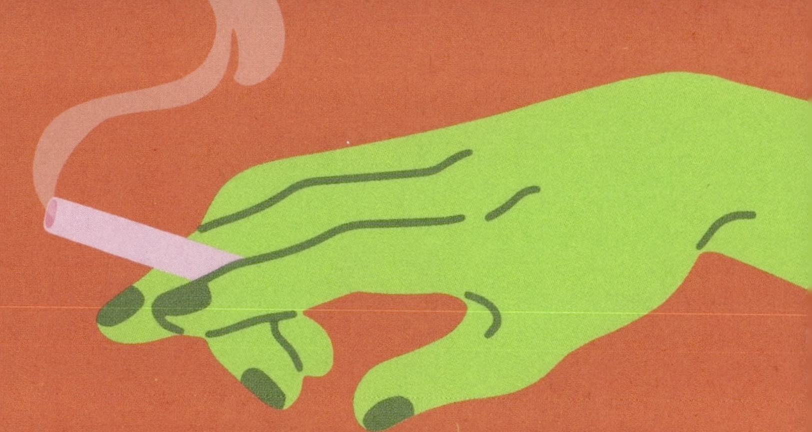

High Activities:
Best Practices for Solo, Couple, and Group Seshes

Creating Joyful Experiences:
Tips for Infusing Daily Life with Mindful Cannabis Consumption

The Ultimate Pairing Guide:
Matching Different Cannabis Forms with Activities

Choose-Your-Own-Adventure Chart

High Activities

Best Practices for Solo, Couple, and Group Seshes

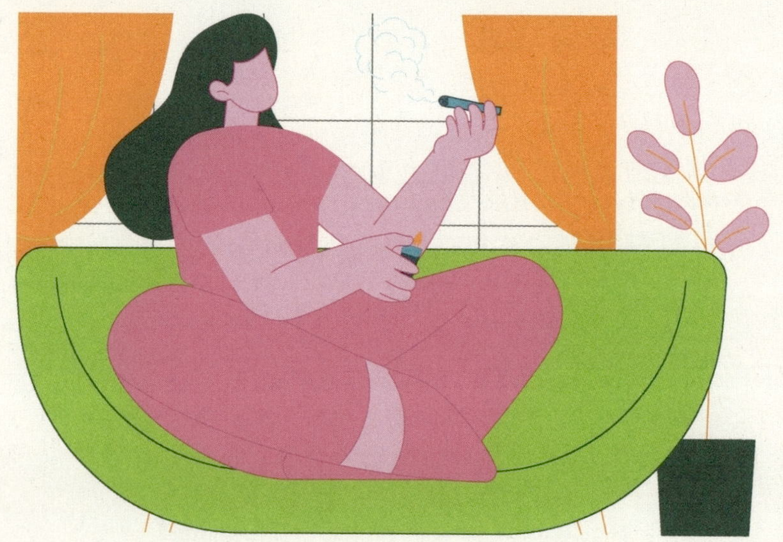

Solo Sesh

Enjoying Your Own Company

Sometimes, the best company is yourself, and a solo sesh can be an ideal way to relax, recharge, and explore new ideas. Here's how to elevate those solo moments.

Set the Mood

Creating a comfortable environment is key to a successful solo sesh. Start by lighting a candle, turning on a favorite lo-fi playlist, or even queuing up an audiobook to transport you to a more relaxed atmosphere. Surround yourself with comfy pillows, and, if possible, dim "the big light"—let candles or softer lamps provide a soothing ambiance instead. One of our favorite ways to unwind is to draw a warm bath. The gentle aroma of some bath salts, combined with the calm, flickering light of a candle, can instantly melt away stress, turning your bath into a true solo spa experience.

Creative Pursuits

Cannabis often has a way of sparking creativity! This is a great time to tap into your artistic side, whether you're painting, drawing, or writing. Adult coloring books are also a fun and nostalgic way to ease into a creative flow without any pressure. We find that a light smoke before editing content helps us focus and stay engaged, especially when staring at a computer screen for long hours. A little dose of inspiration from cannabis can transform an ordinary solo evening into a productive and imaginative session, helping you explore new ideas and expression.

Get Outside

If you prefer to be outdoors, consider taking a walk in nature or setting up a picnic blanket in your backyard. The fresh air, natural sounds, and sights can provide a grounding and rejuvenating high. Moving to Seattle from Los Angeles offered us the chance to experience a larger outdoor space. Alice, for instance, became a passionate bird-watcher in our new neighborhood. She started capturing photos of the birds she spotted and saved them in a dedicated album on her phone. Engaging in little hobbies like this can add a unique element to your outdoor sesh, enhancing your connection to nature.

Mindful Meditation

Practicing mindfulness or meditation with cannabis can deepen your relaxation and focus, helping you clear your mind and find inner peace. Sometimes, it can even turn into a much-needed nap (no shame—we've been there!). If you're new to meditation, YouTube is a great resource, offering guided sessions for all experience levels. Take a few deep breaths, embrace the quiet, and let cannabis help ease you into a more mindful, present state.

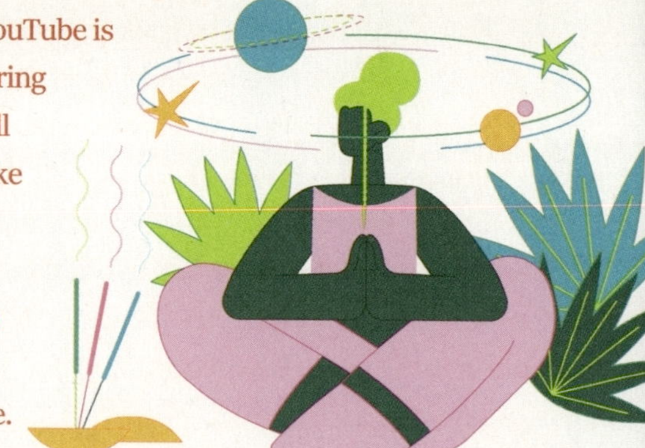

Couple Sesh

Bonding and Connecting

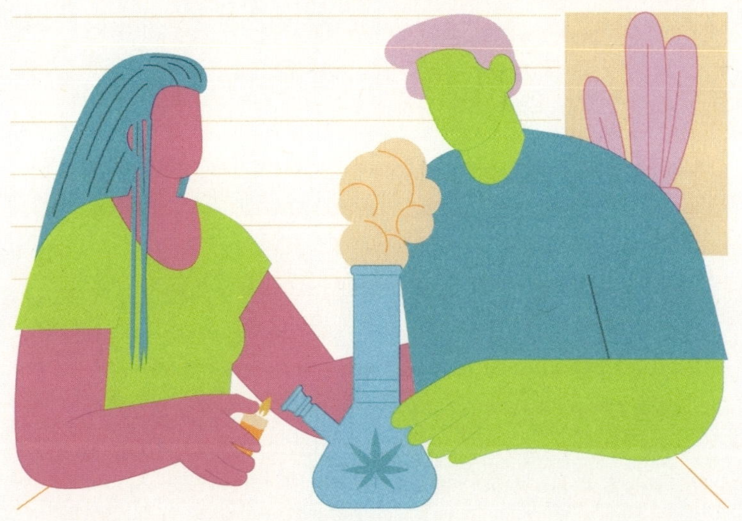

Sharing a cannabis experience with your partner can add a whole new dimension to your relationship. Here's how to make it special:

Choose the Right Strain

Selecting a strain that appeals to both of you can set the tone for your sesh. Indicas are generally more calming and relaxing, perfect for a cozy evening, while Sativas are energizing, helping to spark conversation. Take your time picking a strain that suits both your moods—start with the scent test! Clark and I smoked on our first date, which is a special memory for us, and finding the right strain together now still makes each sesh feel unique.

Cook Together

Cooking together can be a fun, interactive experience that showcases your creativity. We often set up *Chopped*-style challenges, where we each choose three random ingredients from our kitchen and try to create something edible. It's amazing how many delicious munchie creations come out of these impromptu cooking experiments! From wild flavor combinations to the creation of new inside jokes, cooking together with cannabis adds a new layer of connection.

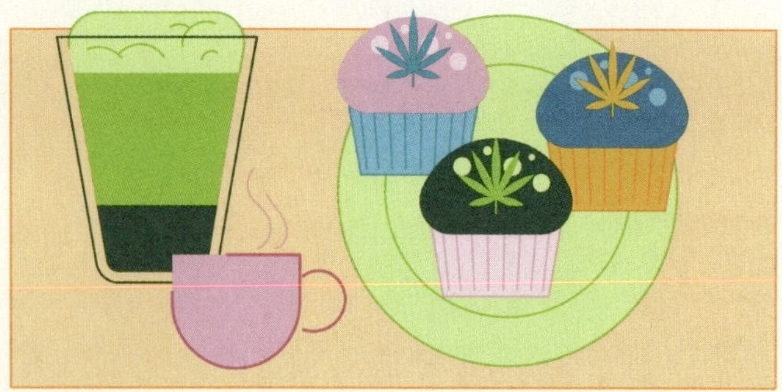

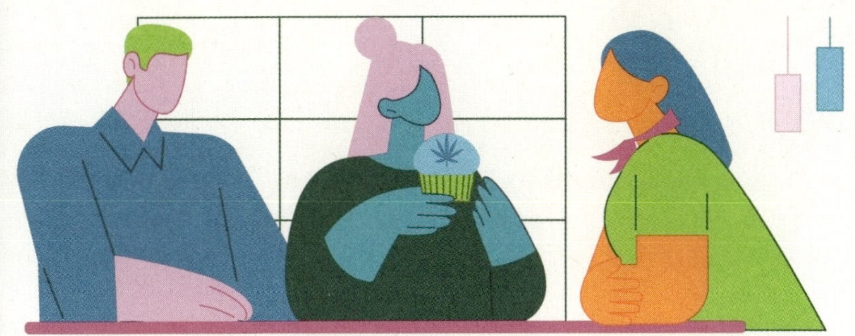

Watch a Movie or Show

Decide on a movie or series before you smoke; choosing what to watch afterward might turn into a blackhole debate. Some of our favorite movies to watch high include *Scott Pilgrim Versus the World*, *Doctor Strange*, *Across the Universe*, *Rango* (the movie we watched on our first date), *Spiderman: Into the Spiderverse*, *Dazed and Confused*, *The Secret Life of Walter Mitty*, *The Grand Budapest Hotel*, *Her*, and pretty much any nature documentary made in the last twenty years.

Deep Conversations

Cannabis has a way of opening new levels of conversation. Whether you're sharing funny stories or discussing dreams and goals, a little cannabis can encourage honesty and vulnerability. Here are fifteen fun conversation starters to ask your partner while seshing together:

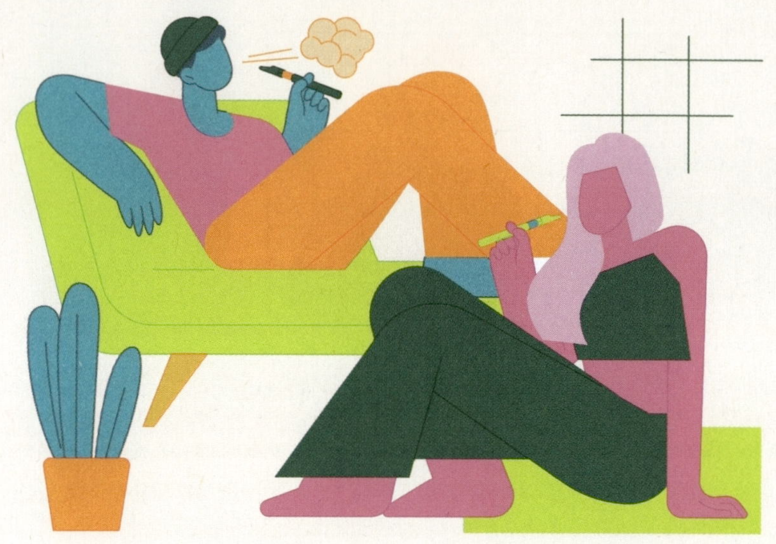

1. If you could **relive any moment** from your past, what would it be and why?

2. What's your **favorite memory** of us together?

3. Is there a **place** you've always wanted to visit?

4. If you could only eat **one meal** for the rest of your life, what would it be?

5. What's a **story from your childhood** that still makes you laugh?

6. If you **won the lottery tomorrow**, what's the first thing you would do?
7. What's the **weirdest food** you've ever tried, and would you eat it again?
8. If you could be any **fictional character** for a day, who would you be and why?
9. If you could have any **superpower**, what would it be and how would you use it?
10. What would your **dream house** look like, and where would it be located?
11. If you could instantly become an **expert in anything**, what would it be?
12. What's the **most ridiculous thing** you've ever done on a dare?
13. If our life were a movie, **what genre** would it be and who would play us?
14. If you could **sesh with any three people**, dead or alive, who would they be and why?
15. What's your **ultimate road trip destination** and what stops would we make along the way?

Group Sesh

Fun with Friends

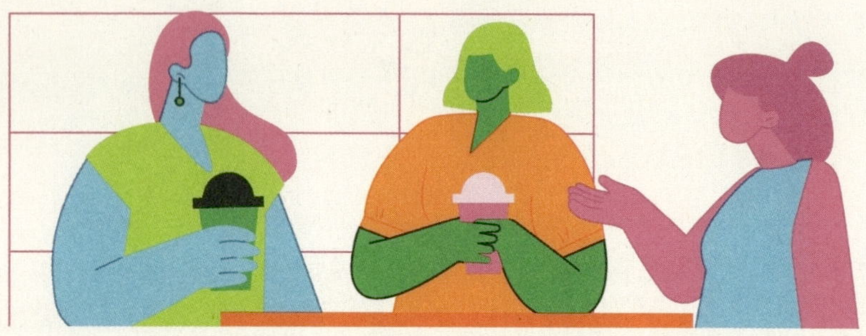

When you're friends with Mary Jane, every gathering is more enjoyable. Here are a few best practices for every experience level.

Set Ground Rules

Before you begin, make sure everyone is comfortable and aware of each other's boundaries. Not everyone has the same tolerance or preference for cannabis, so avoid any unspoken "hit-for-hit" expectations and emphasize that everyone should feel comfortable saying no. Respect each person's experience level to make sure that everyone has a good time.

Play Games

Cannabis and games are a classic pairing, adding humor and competition to the sesh. Board games and video games alike create a lively atmosphere—some of our favorite picks are Mario Kart 8, UNO, and Jackbox Party Pack. Games are fantastic for building memories with friends, whether it's your tenth or one hundredth group sesh together.

Enjoy Music

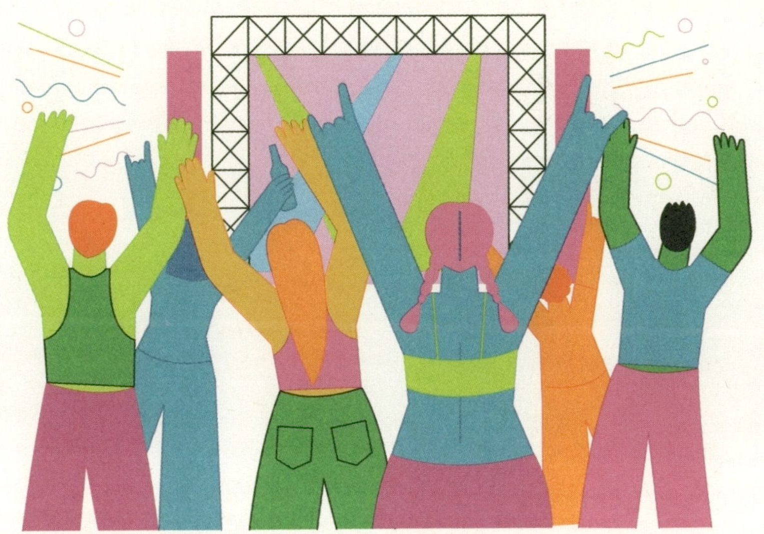

Music naturally enhances any cannabis experience. For those who enjoy concerts, remember to be respectful of venue rules. We learned the hard way when trying to light up during a Wiz Khalifa concert at the Hollywood Bowl—it turns out not even outdoor venues are always 420-friendly. For those staying in, create a playlist or take turns as DJ. Music has always been an easy window into someone's personality and there's nothing quite like a hotbox car karaoke sesh.

Try a New Activity Together

It can be easier to try something new as a group because you know you have the support of your friends, including Mary Jane. This could be anything from a creative workshop to a hike to volunteering to help your community. Experiencing new things together, while a little stoned, strengthens bonds and is bound to create a new inside joke or two. When we lived in California we'd love to get a good group of friends together and rent a cabin out in the woods for a long weekend. Not everyone would know each other before the trip, but everyone would bring something new to the table for fun that weekend. Making sure we always had something on hand to sesh with elevated the overall vibe of the weekend.

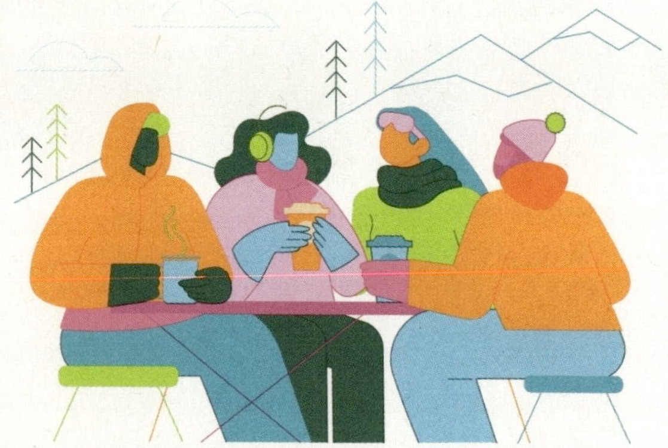

Best Practices for All Seshes

- **Stay Hydrated**—Keep water or a hydrating drink nearby. Cannabis is known to cause dry mouth, and staying hydrated is key to a comfortable experience.
- **Have Snacks Ready**—Prepare some snacks ahead of time. Having munchies on hand can make your sesh more enjoyable and keep hunger at bay.
- **Know Your Limits**—Be mindful of your cannabis consumption. Everyone's tolerance is different, so know your limits and respect them to ensure a good time for all, especially if you're trying something new.
- **Create a Safe Space**—Whether you're alone or with others, make sure your environment feels safe and comfortable. A cozy environment can set the tone for the entire sesh.

Remember, the goal is to enjoy and enhance your time with cannabis, whether you're alone, with a partner, or in a group. Stay lifted, stay happy, and make the most of every sesh!

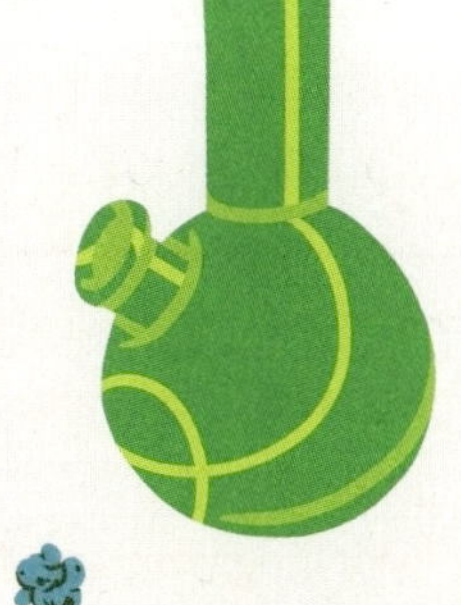

Creating Joyful Experiences

Tips for Infusing Daily Life with Mindful Cannabis Consumption

Lots of people believe that daily cannabis consumption is a slippery slope to becoming the "lazy stoner" stereotype often seen in pop culture, but it's about building habits. If you consume cannabis with intention you'll see how much it can enhance instead of inhibit. Incorporating cannabis into your daily routine can transform ordinary activities into intentional moments of joy and presence. It's about enhancing your experiences, not escaping from life, and using cannabis to create positive energy and deeper connections.

Start Your Day with Intention

Begin your day with a mindful approach. Setting a positive tone in the morning, with a wake-and-bake alongside some eggs and bacon, can put you in the right headspace. For a morning meditation, consider a small dose of a Sativa-dominant strain, like Tangerine Dream, to energize and focus your mind: This little hit beats a morning latte any day. For those who enjoy movement, light stretching or yoga with an energizing strain can make the morning routine feel refreshing and focused. If you're not sure where to start, free yoga routines on social media are an easy way to get going.

Enhance Your Meals

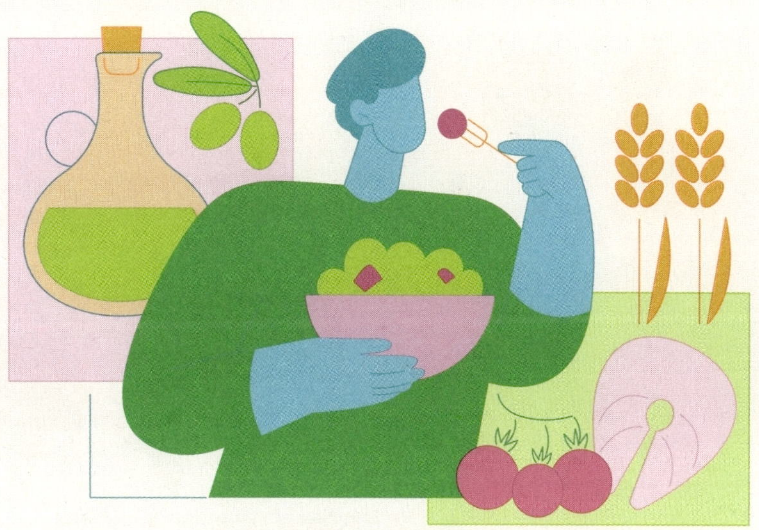

Cannabis can turn a simple meal into a mindful and delightful experience. Think of each dish as a work of art you're about to savor. One way to start experimenting is with infused cooking: add small amounts of cannabis oil or butter to dishes like oven-baked desserts or salad dressings. Remember to go slow with edibles—you can always add more, but you can't take it back. Cannabis can also heighten your senses and make you more aware of flavors and textures. Try exploring new combinations; if you love sweet and sour, you might enjoy pairing sweet and spicy. Some of our classic favorites for this are grilled cheese, air-fryer chicken wings, and, of course, doughnuts.

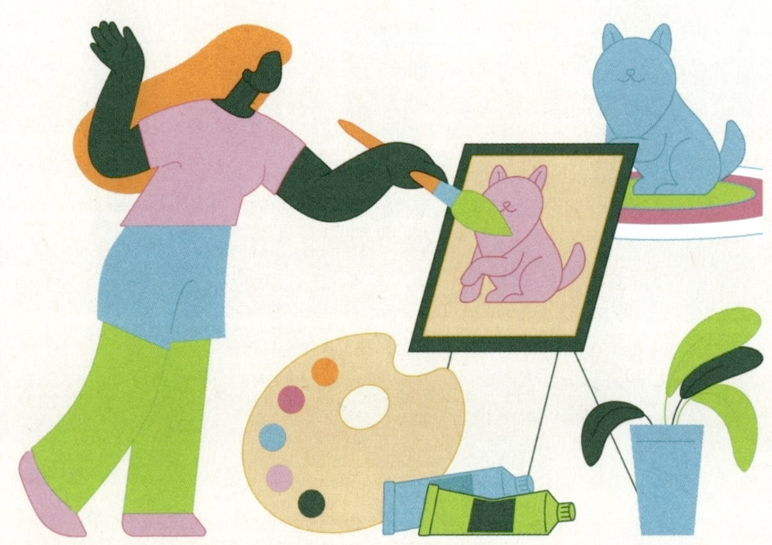

Incorporate Cannabis into Creative Projects

Cannabis has a reputation for sparking creativity, and it's played a huge part in our creative lives, especially in building our social brand, That High Couple. It's the fuel that keeps us inspired and motivated even through the more mundane aspects of the creative process. If you're diving into a creative session, a balanced hybrid strain can provide relaxation without losing focus, making it great for painting, writing, or crafting. We're high right now writing this book! Cannabis can also deepen your appreciation for music or visual art, letting you explore new ideas and inspirations. Some of our favorite artists to enjoy while high include David Bowie, Alt-J, Gorillaz, Action Bronson, Tame Impala, Florence + the Machine, and pretty much any John Williams soundtrack.

Elevate Your Workouts

For those who enjoy movement, cannabis can make physical activities more engaging and fun. Even if you're at home, pairing cannabis with your workout routine can help you stay motivated. A Sativa strain or edible before exercise can give you that extra push to get moving. We love munching on gummies before heading to the gym—it gives us a positive burst of energy that makes every squat and stretch feel like an accomplishment. To keep the momentum, put together a high-energy playlist for a fun, focused session. And when you're done, a CBD or Indica strain can help soothe sore muscles and make post-workout relaxation even more rewarding. After a tough workout, winding down with a CBD-infused topical and an Indica vape session feels like a well-earned treat.

Create a Relaxing Evening Ritual

As the day winds down, consider using cannabis to help set the stage for a restful night. While Alice can fall asleep almost anywhere, Clark has a harder time, so he's started taking a CBN edible an hour before bed to ease into sleep mode. Creating a consistent, relaxing routine like this can help you drift off more naturally. Brewing a cup of cannabis-infused herbal tea also makes for a cozy evening treat. With a touch of honey and lemon, this warm drink can gently ease you into a calm, peaceful state. For extra relaxation, try combining a cannabis-infused bath bomb with some lavender or eucalyptus oil for an aromatic bath–Alice swears by it for winding down.

Enhance Social Connections

Cannabis has a natural way of bringing people together. Whether it's at a social gathering or simply hanging out with friends, sharing a joint can open conversations and make laughter come more easily. Over the years, we've met some of our best friends at cannabis events, where everyone is more open and eager to connect. Alice always has a pre-roll or vape in her purse, ready to share whenever the moment strikes. For couples, a sesh together can be a beautiful way to bond, whether you're doing an activity or sharing a quiet moment. There's something about sharing cannabis that strengthens connections, making it easy to feel close and present.

Practice Mindful Consumption

Ultimately, the key to positive cannabis experiences is mindful consumption. Pay attention to how different strains and doses make you feel, and try to use cannabis with a purpose. Keeping a journal—Clark just uses the Notes app on his phone—can help you track which strains work best for certain activities, allowing you to discover what enhances your experiences. When you're consuming, stay present. Focus on each flavor and aroma, take deep breaths, and allow yourself to fully appreciate the moment.

By bringing cannabis into your daily routine with purpose, you're creating opportunities to make each day more meaningful and enjoyable. From morning to night, it's about enhancing your life and creating connections with yourself, others, and the world around you.

The Ultimate Pairing Guide
Matching Different Cannabis Forms with Activities

When it comes to pairing cannabis with activities, there's no rulebook. Everyone's experience is unique, and what works for one person might not work for another. However, after years of experimenting, we've found some ideal pairings based on our experiences that can enhance different activities. Here's a guide to help you find the best cannabis form for your next adventure.

For Social Gatherings: Joints and Blunts

For hanging out with friends, there's no better companion than a joint or a blunt. These classic options are perfect for socializing—shareable, portable, and easy to pass around. If you're in a group and no one has rolling skills, you can always grab a pre-roll from a dispensary or use a cone that's easy to pack yourself (our go-to). Joints and blunts also offer versatility, as you can roll them with different strains to match the vibe of the session. Whether it's a backyard BBQ, a beach party, or a casual get-together, passing around a joint while playing cards, enjoying music, or engaging in deep conversations makes for an effortlessly fun time.

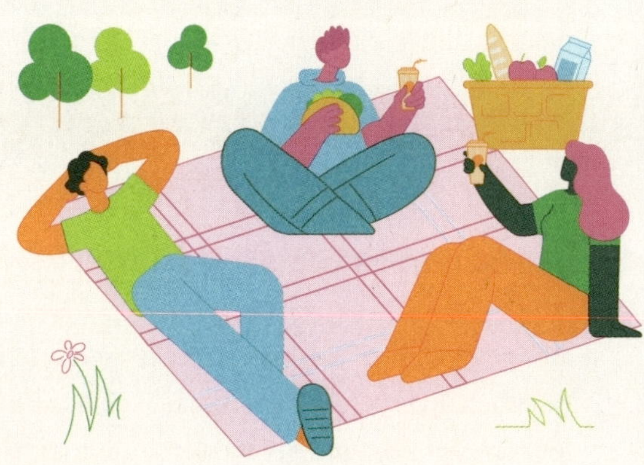

For Hiking: Vape Pens

When you're on a nature trail, a vape pen is an excellent choice. Not only are they discreet and easy to carry, but they're also safer than open flames, making them perfect for outdoor activities. Vape pens offer a controlled dose of cannabis, and we love taking small puffs to manage our high throughout the hike. Whether you're on a scenic trail with breathtaking views or simply enjoying the serenity of the woods, pairing a vape pen with a good playlist or podcast can elevate the experience.

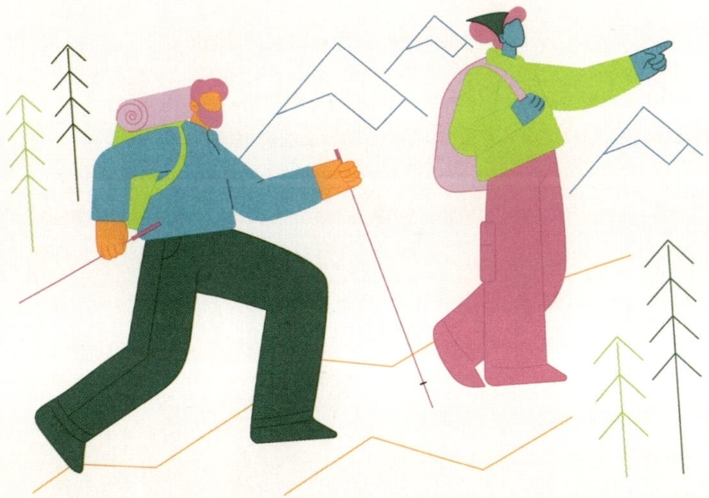

For Movie Nights: Dabs

If you're looking to settle in for a cozy movie night or binge-watching session, dabs are a great way to get fast, powerful effects that will have you fully immersed in whatever you're watching. Dabs are quick-acting and deliver an intense high, which makes them perfect for those who want to relax on the couch without any distractions. Pair dabs with a sci-fi or fantasy film for an enhanced experience or enjoy gourmet snacks like popcorn with unique seasonings or your favorite comfort food while you indulge.

For Creative Projects: Edibles

When you're diving into a creative project, you want something that will keep your mind engaged without interrupting your flow. That's where edibles come in. They offer a long-lasting, steady high, which is ideal for activities like painting, writing, crafting, or playing music. For a smooth creative experience, we recommend taking smaller doses throughout the session rather than one large dose at the start. Whether you're in a well-lit space surrounded by your creative tools or just getting into the zone, edibles can help keep the inspiration flowing for hours.

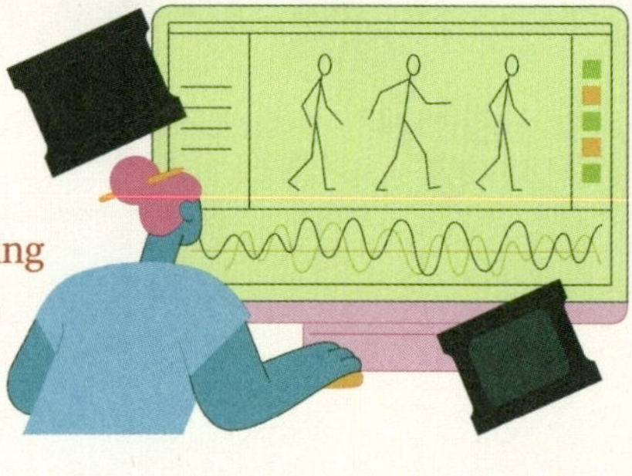

For Meditation and Yoga: Tinctures

For moments of calm and introspection, tinctures provide a controlled and precise dosing experience. Their quick onset, especially when taken sublingually, makes them an excellent choice for activities like meditation and yoga. You can easily adjust the amount of cannabis to match your desired experience, allowing you to focus without being overwhelmed. Pair tinctures with a gentle flow or restorative yoga session or use them to deepen your meditation practice. Whether you're doing guided meditation or enjoying personal reflection time, tinctures can help enhance the tranquility of your practice.

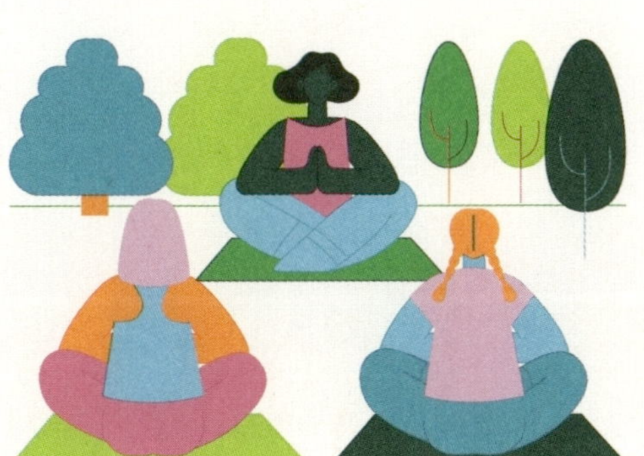

For a Casual Day Out: Flower

When you're out and about for a casual day, traditional flower is always a reliable and versatile option. With so many strains to choose from, you can pick one that suits your mood for whatever activity you have planned. For us, joints or pre-rolls are our go-to for an easy, convenient way to enjoy cannabis while walking around the city, visiting a museum, or enjoying a picnic in the park. Flower pairs perfectly with a portable pipe or one-hitter for convenience, allowing you to enjoy the experience without hassle.

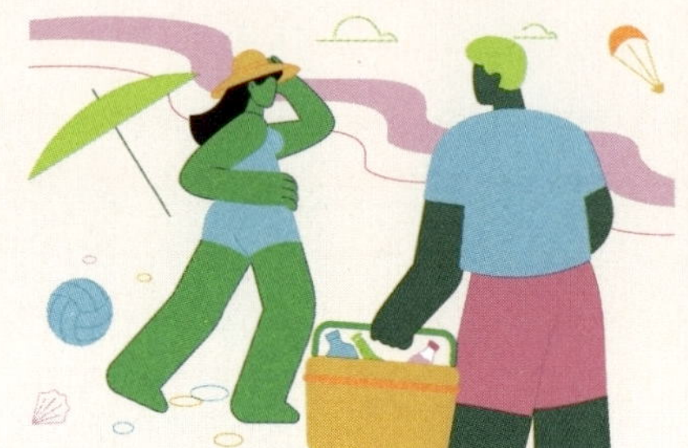

For Deep Relaxation: Topicals

After a long day, the soothing effects of cannabis-infused topicals can help you unwind and relax. These products provide the benefits of cannabis without the high, which makes them perfect for anyone looking to relax their body without feeling impaired. Whether you're soaking in a warm bath, curling up with a good book, or enjoying a massage, topicals can target specific areas of tension and offer a calming experience. With various CBD lotions on hand, it's easy to find the right relief for different needs.

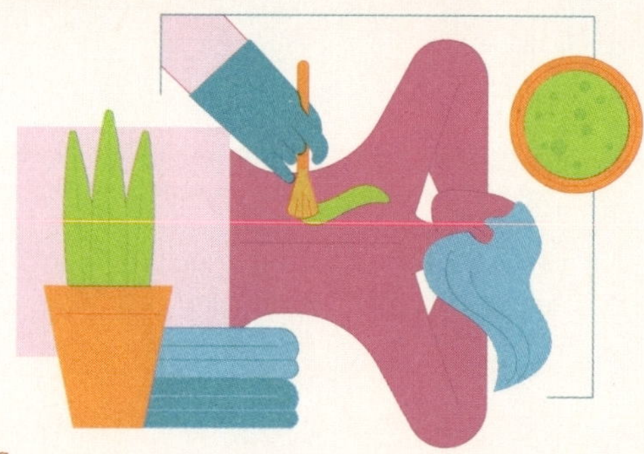

For Gaming: Sativa-Dominant Strains

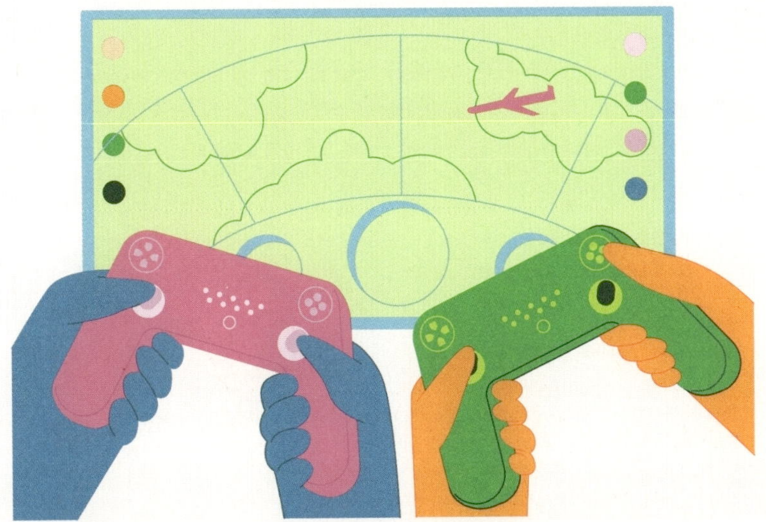

For gaming, whether it's video games or board games, Sativa-dominant strains can keep you engaged and alert. These uplifting and energizing strains are perfect for maintaining focus, improving concentration, and enhancing reaction time. Whether you're racing through a fast-paced video game, solving puzzles, or strategizing in a board game, Sativa strains help keep your mind sharp and the good vibes going.

For Exercising: THC-Infused Beverages

If you enjoy working out, THC-infused beverages can be the perfect pre- or post-workout companion. They provide a mild, manageable high while keeping you hydrated, which is essential during physical activities. These beverages allow you to control the amount of cannabis you consume, ensuring you get just the right amount of relaxation and energy. Whether you're doing yoga, jogging, or hitting the gym, a THC-infused beverage can make your workout more enjoyable, and sipping one during an outdoor activity like hiking or biking can add an extra layer of fun.

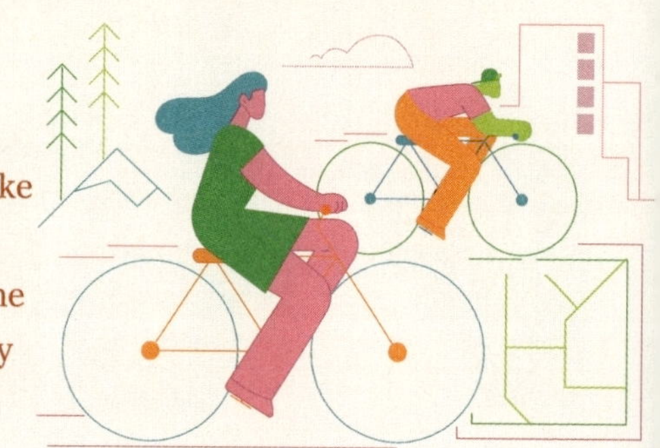

For Gardening: Sun-Grown Flower

For those who love gardening, there's something special about pairing your time in the garden with sun-grown cannabis. The connection between nature and cannabis is deep, and enjoying a strain that has been grown outdoors can enhance the experience. Sun-grown flowers usually offer a mild, pleasant high that pairs perfectly with the earthy, grounding task of gardening. Whether you're planting

flowers, tending to vegetables, or landscaping, enjoy the process with a strain that has been nurtured by the sun. Ask your budtender about outdoor-grown strains for the best selection.

By matching the right form of cannabis with the right activity, you can enhance your experience and get the most out of every moment. Experiment with different pairings, see what works best for you, and enjoy the journey!

Choose-Your-Own-*Adventure* Chart

START HERE:
What kind of vibe are you in the mood for?

Relaxed & Low-Key
→ Option A

Playful & Social
→ Option B

Creative & Inspiring
→ Option C

Option A: *Relaxed & Low-Key*

Solo:

Run a warm bath with a cannabis-infused bath bomb.

Cozy up with a book or an audiobook and a calming Indica strain like Granddaddy Purple.

Couple:

Try a shared guided meditation or slow yoga flow with a hybrid strain like Blue Dream.

End the evening with a cannabis-infused massage oil and relaxing music.

Group:

Host a "Zen Night" with friends—think CBD teas, light conversation, and candles.

Watch a nature documentary with a mellow strain like Harlequin.

Option B: *Playful & Social*

Solo:

Test your cooking skills by whipping up an infused snack.

Try a video game or watch a nostalgic movie with a balanced strain like Gelato.

Couple:

Try making homemade infused pizzas—choose your toppings and create a flavor masterpiece together.

Watch a rom-com or play board games with an uplifting strain like Lemon Haze.

Group:

Organize a game night with classics like Clue or a multiplayer video game.

Have a karaoke night—pick your favorite songs, grab a mic (or a hairbrush), and sing your heart out!

Option C:
Creative & Inspiring

Solo:

Start a new art project (painting, drawing, or crafting).

Take a walk in nature or write poetry with a Sativa strain like Jack Herer.

Couple:

Plan a vision-board session with old magazines and scissors.

Take a sunset hike together with a strain like Super Silver Haze.

Group:

Host a "Paint and Sesh" night. Provide supplies like canvases and paints.

Try an open-mic session where everyone shares stories, songs, or poems while enjoying a creative strain like Tangie.

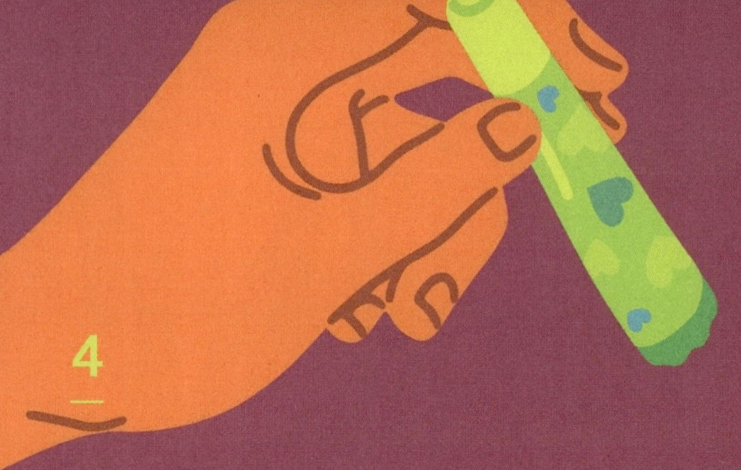

4

Relationship Bliss *Through* Cannabis

With Significant Others: Integrating Cannabis into Your Romantic Life

Discussing Cannabis with a Partner Who Doesn't Consume

With Significant Others

Integrating Cannabis into Your Romantic Life

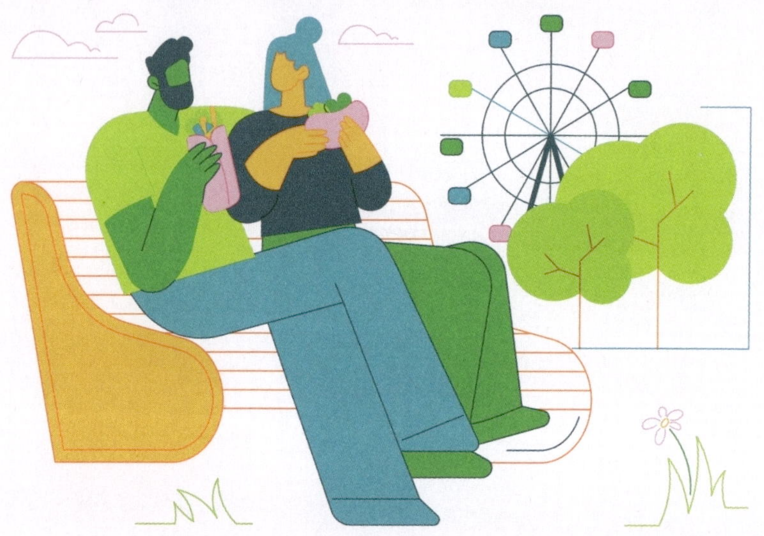

As That High Couple, we've always believed that cannabis can be a wonderful addition to your romantic life. It has the power to elevate date nights, enhance intimacy, and create unique experiences. We're especially excited to dive into this chapter because we have many ways cannabis can be integrated into your relationship.

One of the simplest ways to enhance a date is by sharing cannabis together. Whether you light a joint or enjoy an edible, the shared experience of getting elevated can help set a fun and relaxed mood. It's important to plan your activities around the idea of being high, but you don't have to go overboard with fancy plans or extravagant costs. A date can be anything you both enjoy doing together—whether it's a spontaneous adventure or a thoughtful activity. A great starting point is something as simple as sharing a pre-roll while on a walk or enjoying a sunset. From there, let the experience unfold. We've had some of the best memories from uncomplicated dates that turned into extraordinary moments just by adding a little cannabis into the mix.

For daytime dates, we've enjoyed everything from visiting art galleries to having a laid-back picnic at the park. If you're looking for something more unique, check out your local botanical garden or aquarium or even visit a farmers market to sample some local foods. If you're more into creative activities, pottery classes or cooking together can be fun while elevated—adding cannabis to these experiences can make them more relaxed and enjoyable.

For nighttime dates, we've always been fans of concerts or stargazing while high. Something about the music or the vast sky feels more magical when you're in the right state of mind. We've also had a blast attending comedy shows or enjoying an evening at the beach with a bonfire, sharing a joint and watching the flames dance. If you're looking for a cozy night in, try making an ice cream bar with all your favorite toppings while enjoying edibles. The possibilities are endless, and cannabis can make even the simplest activities feel like a celebration of your time together.

When you've been in a relationship for a while, it's easy to feel like you've explored every local date idea. That's when ongoing date ideas come into play. One thing we love doing is creating a food truck bracket, where we try different trucks in the city and rank our favorites. We also enjoy going on walks and cataloging the local plants or birds we see, turning a simple walk into a fun, shared activity. One of our more recent ongoing ideas is getting flowers from the local grocery store and having a monthly challenge to see who can create the better bouquet (Clark always wins!). These simple activities, when combined with cannabis, create lasting memories and help us feel connected.

Cannabis also plays a big role in enhancing intimacy in our relationship. It helps us feel more relaxed and present with each other, creating the perfect environment for deeper emotional and physical connections. A great way to set the mood is by creating a calming atmosphere–light some candles, play soft music, and use aromatherapy to help foster relaxation. Sharing a joint or an edible can be part of this ritual, helping both partners relax and create a deeper bond.

Cannabis can also help ease any anxiety around intimacy. For those who feel nervous or stressed in intimate situations, cannabis can be a game-changer. It helps us relax, clear our minds, and open to each other in ways that might not have been possible without it. One of our most profound experiences has been using cannabis to deepen our emotional connection. It's amazing how cannabis can help facilitate meaningful conversations where we express feelings we may have been holding back. It's not just about getting high–it's about creating a space to be open, truly listen, and connect on a deeper level.

To take intimacy to the next level, we've found that cannabis-infused products like massage oils, lubricants, and bath bombs can enhance the experience. Cannabis-infused massage oils, for example, help relax muscles and relieve tension, making massages feel more soothing. And if you're looking to heighten physical intimacy, cannabis-infused lubricants can increase sensitivity, making the experience more enjoyable for both partners. These products are fantastic because they're topically applied, so they don't give you a psychoactive effect, but they do bring added pleasure to the physical sensations.

Part of the fun of integrating cannabis into your intimate life is experimenting together. Try different strains, dosages, and consumption methods to see what works best for you both. Some nights, we love a relaxing Indica to unwind before bed, while other times, a playful Sativa sets the mood for an afternoon adventure. What's most important is to communicate openly about how each of you is feeling and to keep experimenting until you find your sweet spot as a couple.

Discussing Cannabis with a Partner Who Doesn't Consume

Talking about cannabis with a partner who doesn't consume can feel tricky, but it doesn't have to be. The key is to approach the conversation with understanding, empathy, and respect. Choosing the right time and place to initiate this discussion is critical. You don't want to bring it up in the middle of an argument or when your partner is stressed. Instead, wait for a calm moment where you can both engage in an open, uninterrupted conversation.

Educating your partner about cannabis is a great way to start. They may have misconceptions or concerns and presenting them with accurate information can help alleviate those worries. Explain how cannabis benefits you personally—whether it helps you relax, reduces stress, or enhances your creativity. Share the positive impact it has had on your well-being and why it's something you choose to incorporate into your life.

Honesty is key when explaining why cannabis is important to you. Be open about how it positively impacts your life, and make sure to express your willingness to respect their perspective as well. It's essential to listen to your partner's concerns with an open mind. Perhaps they have reservations about the legality of cannabis, its health effects, or its social stigma. Acknowledge their feelings and provide reassurances where possible but also remain patient if they need time to process the information.

Discussing boundaries is another important aspect. If your partner is uncomfortable with cannabis use in certain spaces or at certain times, be open to compromise. Maybe they're okay with you smoking outside or consuming edibles privately. The goal is to ensure that both of you are comfortable with the arrangement and you respect each other's boundaries.

If your partner is open to learning more about cannabis but doesn't consume it, involve them in non-consumption activities. Take them to a dispensary or attend a cannabis-related event together. Watching an educational documentary can also be a good way to demystify cannabis, making it feel less intimidating. The key is to show them that you're not trying to push cannabis use onto them but simply want them to understand it better.

Finally, it's important to be patient and understanding. Changing someone's perspective on cannabis takes time, and it may take several conversations before your partner fully understands why it's important to you. Continue to reassure them that their comfort matters to you and remain open-minded as they process their thoughts. If the conversation continues to create tension, seeking guidance from a couple's therapist can help provide a neutral space to resolve any lingering concerns.

By approaching the conversation with respect, openness, and patience, you can navigate any differences and work toward a better understanding of cannabis in your relationship. This dialogue can strengthen your connection, enhance mutual respect, and ensure that both partners feel heard and supported.

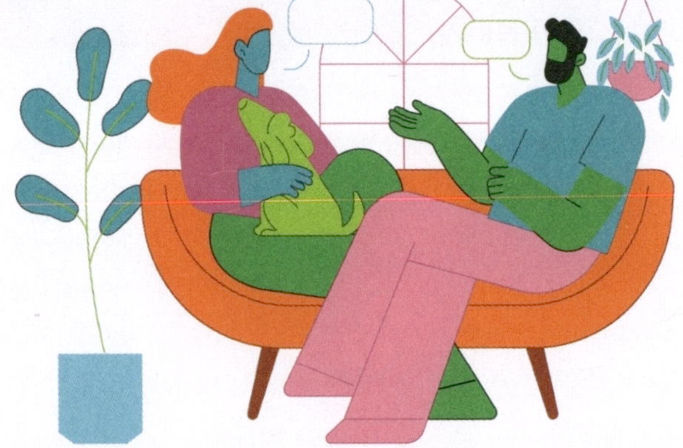

Cannabis Date Night Planner

What's the vibe for the night? *(Circle one or more):*	
Cozy and intimate	Relaxing and restorative
Fun and playful	Adventurous and active
Creative and artsy	Other:
Choose your strain: *(Circle one):*	
Indica (relax and unwind)	
Sativa (energize and uplift)	
Hybrid (a balanced mix)	
What's the activity? *(Circle one or more):*	
Movie night at home	Cooking or baking together
Art project or DIY crafting	Picnic under the stars
Walk or hike in nature	Other:

<table>
<tr><td colspan="2">Set the scene:
(Fill in with some ideas that you'll enjoy)</td></tr>
<tr><td colspan="2">Snacks or food to prepare:</td></tr>
<tr><td colspan="2">Music or playlist:</td></tr>
<tr><td colspan="2">Lighting or décor:</td></tr>
<tr><td colspan="2">How will you consume cannabis?
(Circle one):</td></tr>
<tr><td>Pre-rolls or joints</td><td>Edibles or infused drinks</td></tr>
<tr><td>Tinctures or oils</td><td>Other:</td></tr>
</table>

Reflect on the experience:

What was your favorite part of the night?

What would you do differently next time?

How did cannabis enhance your time together?

What's the vibe for the night? *(Circle one or more):*	
Cozy and intimate	Relaxing and restorative
Fun and playful	Adventurous and active
Creative and artsy	Other:
Choose your strain: *(Circle one):*	
Indica (relax and unwind)	
Sativa (energize and uplift)	
Hybrid (a balanced mix)	
What's the activity? *(Circle one or more):*	
Movie night at home	Cooking or baking together
Art project or DIY crafting	Picnic under the stars
Walk or hike in nature	Other:
Set the scene: *(Fill in with some ideas that you'll enjoy)*	
Snacks or food to prepare:	
Music or playlist:	

Lighting or décor:	
How will you consume cannabis? *(Circle one):*	
Pre-rolls or joints	Edibles or infused drinks
Tinctures or oils	Other:

Reflect on the experience:

What was your favorite part of the night?

What would you do differently next time?

How did cannabis enhance your time together?

<table>
<tr><th colspan="2">What's the vibe for the night?
(Circle one or more):</th></tr>
<tr><td>Cozy and intimate</td><td>Relaxing and restorative</td></tr>
<tr><td>Fun and playful</td><td>Adventurous and active</td></tr>
<tr><td>Creative and artsy</td><td>Other:</td></tr>
<tr><th colspan="2">Choose your strain:
(Circle one):</th></tr>
<tr><td colspan="2">Indica (relax and unwind)</td></tr>
<tr><td colspan="2">Sativa (energize and uplift)</td></tr>
<tr><td colspan="2">Hybrid (a balanced mix)</td></tr>
<tr><th colspan="2">What's the activity?
(Circle one or more):</th></tr>
<tr><td>Movie night at home</td><td>Cooking or baking together</td></tr>
<tr><td>Art project or DIY crafting</td><td>Picnic under the stars</td></tr>
<tr><td>Walk or hike in nature</td><td>Other:</td></tr>
<tr><th colspan="2">Set the scene:
(Fill in with some ideas that you'll enjoy)</th></tr>
<tr><td colspan="2">Snacks or food to prepare:</td></tr>
<tr><td colspan="2">Music or playlist:</td></tr>
</table>

Lighting or décor:	
How will you consume cannabis? *(Circle one):*	
Pre-rolls or joints	Edibles or infused drinks
Tinctures or oils	Other:

Reflect on the experience:

What was your favorite part of the night?

What would you do differently next time?

How did cannabis enhance your time together?

What's the vibe for the night? *(Circle one or more):*	
Cozy and intimate	Relaxing and restorative
Fun and playful	Adventurous and active
Creative and artsy	Other:

Choose your strain: *(Circle one):*
Indica (relax and unwind)
Sativa (energize and uplift)
Hybrid (a balanced mix)

What's the activity? *(Circle one or more):*	
Movie night at home	Cooking or baking together
Art project or DIY crafting	Picnic under the stars
Walk or hike in nature	Other:

Set the scene: *(Fill in with some ideas that you'll enjoy)*
Snacks or food to prepare:
Music or playlist:

<table>
<tr><td colspan="2">Lighting or décor:</td></tr>
<tr><td colspan="2">How will you consume cannabis?
(Circle one):</td></tr>
<tr><td>Pre-rolls or joints</td><td>Edibles or infused drinks</td></tr>
<tr><td>Tinctures or oils</td><td>Other:</td></tr>
</table>

Reflect on the experience:

What was your favorite part of the night?

What would you do differently next time?

How did cannabis enhance your time together?

What's the vibe for the night? *(Circle one or more):*	
Cozy and intimate	Relaxing and restorative
Fun and playful	Adventurous and active
Creative and artsy	Other:

Choose your strain: *(Circle one):*
Indica (relax and unwind)
Sativa (energize and uplift)
Hybrid (a balanced mix)

What's the activity? *(Circle one or more):*	
Movie night at home	Cooking or baking together
Art project or DIY crafting	Picnic under the stars
Walk or hike in nature	Other:

Set the scene: *(Fill in with some ideas that you'll enjoy)*
Snacks or food to prepare:
Music or playlist:

Lighting or décor:	
How will you consume cannabis? *(Circle one):*	
Pre-rolls or joints	Edibles or infused drinks
Tinctures or oils	Other:

Reflect on the experience:

What was your favorite part of the night?

What would you do differently next time?

How did cannabis enhance your time together?

With Family

How to Discuss Cannabis with Your Family, and Sharing a Sesh with Relatives

Discussing cannabis with family members can be just as sensitive as talking to a partner who doesn't consume it. However, it's an important step toward fostering understanding and reducing stigma. As with any tough conversation, it's best to approach it with care and respect. Start by educating yourself about cannabis and its benefits so you can provide accurate information when discussing it with your family. Whether it's for wellness, relaxation, or pain management, showing them how cannabis positively impacts your life can make them more open to the idea.

Starting the dialogue honestly and openly is key. Explain why you choose to use cannabis and listen to their concerns. Be sure to emphasize that responsible use is important to you and that it's a personal choice that doesn't negatively affect your relationship with them. If they're open to it, you can even share a cannabis session together, starting with something mild like a CBD-dominant strain or a low-dose edible. Creating a relaxed environment and engaging in simple activities like playing board games or watching a movie can help everyone feel comfortable and ease into the experience.

If your family is hesitant, be patient and respectful of their views. With time, they may come to see cannabis in a new light. Just as with a partner, be open to revisiting the conversation and reaffirming your commitment to a healthy, respectful relationship, whether they fully understand your cannabis use or not.

Cannabis and Family Connections Tracker

Use the charts on the next few pages to log moments of shared understanding and positive cannabis experiences with family members. Examples of family-friendly activities could include watching a movie together while enjoying CBD edibles, preparing a cannabis-infused meal together, or sharing stories about your cannabis journey in a relaxed setting.

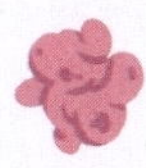

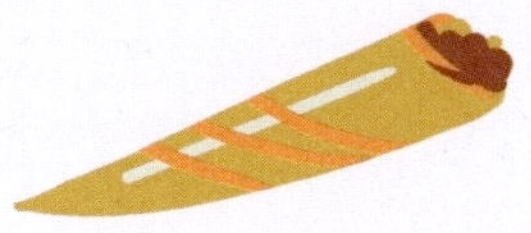

Date	Family Member(s)	Activity/ Topic	What Worked Well	What I'd Change Next Time

Date	Family Member(s)	Activity/ Topic	What Worked Well	What I'd Change Next Time

Date	Family Member(s)	Activity/ Topic	What Worked Well	What I'd Change Next Time

With Friends

Selecting Activities and Conversation Topics for Social Sessions

Cannabis has the power to elevate social interactions, turning ordinary meetups with friends into something memorable and deeply enjoyable. Whether you're looking to keep things lighthearted or dive into more meaningful conversations, cannabis can enhance your time together, making each moment feel more vibrant and relaxed. From casual hangouts to more organized events, there are countless ways to integrate cannabis into your social gatherings, enriching the experience and deepening your connection with friends.

When it comes to activities, the key is to choose those that are easygoing and engaging, allowing everyone to be present and enjoy the moment. A cannabis-infused dinner party is one great way to combine food and cannabis in a fun and sophisticated way. Imagine sharing a multicourse meal where each dish is thoughtfully infused, creating a playful atmosphere that encourages laughter, experimentation, and, of course, delicious conversation. Cooking together, or even enjoying a meal prepared by someone else, becomes a shared experience that enhances the enjoyment of the food and the company.

For a more creative twist, you might consider organizing a craft night where everyone can get in touch with their artistic side. Activities like decorating lighters, designing personalized rolling trays, or hosting a "paint and sesh" night can inspire both creativity and connection. Cannabis can help break down barriers, allowing everyone to feel free to express themselves and create something fun. These kinds of activities are perfect for sparking conversation and laughter while indulging in some playful creativity.

If you and your friends enjoy nature, a hike can be a fantastic way to experience the outdoors while also elevating your connection. With a discreet vape pen, you can keep the experience casual and simple, enjoying the peaceful beauty of nature while the effects of cannabis enhance your sense of relaxation and enjoyment. Walking through the outdoors while elevated can feel meditative, making the time spent with friends more rewarding.

Cannabis also has a way of turning conversations into something deeper and more meaningful. When shared among friends, cannabis encourages openness, often leading to richer, more engaging exchanges. Personal stories about your experiences with cannabis can become a fun and revealing way to bond. Talking about the first time you tried cannabis or sharing funny, memorable moments from past sessions can spark a sense of camaraderie and laughter. These conversations also provide an opportunity to talk about your favorite strains or ways to use cannabis—whether it's the calming effects of an edible or the full-faced buzz of a concentrate dab, discussing how different products affect you can lead to interesting insights and recommendations for future sessions.

Beyond casual conversation, cannabis can also inspire more philosophical or creative dialogues. When elevated, the mind often wanders into new territories, and what might begin as a light conversation can evolve into a deeper, more thought-provoking discussion. Whether you're discussing life's big questions, brainstorming creative ideas, or exploring different perspectives, cannabis can open the door to conversations that are both enlightening and enjoyable.

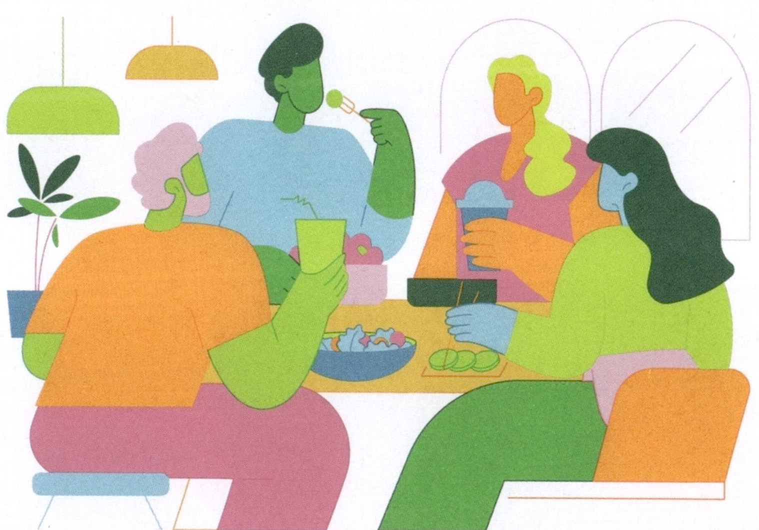

Cannabis Party Checklist

Before the Party	
Choose a theme: *(Examples: "Retro Stoner Night," "Edibles Tasting Party," "Outdoor Sesh in the Park")*	
Curate a playlist:	
Plan the vibe:	
Lighting (candles, fairy lights, etc.)	
Seating (comfy couches, cushions, or bean bags)	
Décor (greenery, fun cannabis-themed touches like leaf-shaped coasters)	
Cannabis Essentials	
Pre-rolls or joints	A mix of Sativa, Indica, and hybrid strains
Edibles (gummies, chocolates, or baked goods)	Vape pens or cartridges
CBD options for those who prefer	Non-psychoactive effects
Smoking accessories (pipes, lighters, rolling papers, grinders)	

<table>
<tr><th colspan="2">Snacks and Drinks</th></tr>
<tr><td colspan="2">Sweet options:</td></tr>
<tr><td colspan="2">Savory options:</td></tr>
<tr><td colspan="2">Non-infused drinks:</td></tr>
<tr><td colspan="2">Infused mocktails or teas (optional):</td></tr>
<tr><th colspan="2">Activities and Games</th></tr>
<tr><td>Classic board games (like Jenga or Uno)</td><td>Video games (Mario Kart, Jackbox)</td></tr>
<tr><td>Art station (paint, doodle pads, clay)</td><td>Music or karaoke setup</td></tr>
<tr><th colspan="2">After the Party</th></tr>
<tr><td colspan="2">What worked well? What could have gone better? How did cannabis enhance the experience?</td></tr>
</table>

Party Report #2

Before the Party	
Choose a theme: *(Examples: "Retro Stoner Night," "Edibles Tasting Party," "Outdoor Sesh in the Park")*	
Curate a playlist:	
Plan the vibe:	
Lighting (candles, fairy lights, etc.)	
Seating (comfy couches, cushions, or bean bags)	
Décor (greenery, fun cannabis-themed touches like leaf-shaped coasters)	
Cannabis Essentials	
Pre-rolls or joints	A mix of Sativa, Indica, and hybrid strains
Edibles (gummies, chocolates, or baked goods)	Vape pens or cartridges
CBD options for those who prefer	Non-psychoactive effects
Smoking accessories (pipes, lighters, rolling papers, grinders)	

Snacks and Drinks	
Sweet options:	
Savory options:	
Non-infused drinks:	
Infused mocktails or teas (optional):	
Activities and Games	
Classic board games (like Jenga or Uno)	Video games (Mario Kart, Jackbox)
Art station (paint, doodle pads, clay)	Music or karaoke setup
After the Party	
What worked well? What could have gone better? How did cannabis enhance the experience?	

Party Report #3

<table>
<tr><th colspan="2">Before the Party</th></tr>
<tr><td colspan="2">Choose a theme: (Examples: "Retro Stoner Night," "Edibles Tasting Party," "Outdoor Sesh in the Park")</td></tr>
<tr><td colspan="2">Curate a playlist:</td></tr>
<tr><td colspan="2">Plan the vibe:</td></tr>
<tr><td colspan="2">Lighting (candles, fairy lights, etc.)</td></tr>
<tr><td colspan="2">Seating (comfy couches, cushions, or bean bags)</td></tr>
<tr><td colspan="2">Décor (greenery, fun cannabis-themed touches like leaf-shaped coasters)</td></tr>
<tr><th colspan="2">Cannabis Essentials</th></tr>
<tr><td>Pre-rolls or joints</td><td>A mix of Sativa, Indica, and hybrid strains</td></tr>
<tr><td>Edibles (gummies, chocolates, or baked goods)</td><td>Vape pens or cartridges</td></tr>
<tr><td>CBD options for those who prefer</td><td>Non-psychoactive effects</td></tr>
<tr><td colspan="2">Smoking accessories (pipes, lighters, rolling papers, grinders)</td></tr>
</table>

<table>
<tr><th colspan="2">Snacks and Drinks</th></tr>
<tr><td colspan="2">Sweet options:</td></tr>
<tr><td colspan="2">Savory options:</td></tr>
<tr><td colspan="2">Non-infused drinks:</td></tr>
<tr><td colspan="2">Infused mocktails or teas (optional):</td></tr>
<tr><th colspan="2">Activities and Games</th></tr>
<tr><td>Classic board games (like Jenga or Uno)</td><td>Video games (Mario Kart, Jackbox)</td></tr>
<tr><td>Art station (paint, doodle pads, clay)</td><td>Music or karaoke setup</td></tr>
<tr><th colspan="2">After the Party</th></tr>
<tr><td colspan="2">What worked well? What could have gone better? How did cannabis enhance the experience?</td></tr>
</table>

Party Report #4

<table>
<tr><th colspan="2">Before the Party</th></tr>
<tr><td colspan="2">Choose a theme: (Examples: “Retro Stoner Night,” “Edibles Tasting Party,” “Outdoor Sesh in the Park”)</td></tr>
<tr><td colspan="2">Curate a playlist:</td></tr>
<tr><td colspan="2">Plan the vibe:</td></tr>
<tr><td colspan="2">Lighting (candles, fairy lights, etc.)</td></tr>
<tr><td colspan="2">Seating (comfy couches, cushions, or bean bags)</td></tr>
<tr><td colspan="2">Décor (greenery, fun cannabis-themed touches like leaf-shaped coasters)</td></tr>
<tr><th colspan="2">Cannabis Essentials</th></tr>
<tr><td>Pre-rolls or joints</td><td>A mix of Sativa, Indica, and hybrid strains</td></tr>
<tr><td>Edibles (gummies, chocolates, or baked goods)</td><td>Vape pens or cartridges</td></tr>
<tr><td>CBD options for those who prefer</td><td>Non-psychoactive effects</td></tr>
<tr><td colspan="2">Smoking accessories (pipes, lighters, rolling papers, grinders)</td></tr>
</table>

Snacks and Drinks	
Sweet options:	
Savory options:	
Non-infused drinks:	
Infused mocktails or teas (optional):	
Activities and Games	
Classic board games (like Jenga or Uno)	Video games (Mario Kart, Jackbox)
Art station (paint, doodle pads, clay)	Music or karaoke setup
After the Party	
What worked well? What could have gone better? How did cannabis enhance the experience?	

Party Report #5

<table>
<tr><th colspan="2">Before the Party</th></tr>
<tr><td colspan="2">Choose a theme: (Examples: "Retro Stoner Night," "Edibles Tasting Party," "Outdoor Sesh in the Park")</td></tr>
<tr><td colspan="2">Curate a playlist:</td></tr>
<tr><td colspan="2">Plan the vibe:</td></tr>
<tr><td colspan="2">Lighting (candles, fairy lights, etc.)</td></tr>
<tr><td colspan="2">Seating (comfy couches, cushions, or bean bags)</td></tr>
<tr><td colspan="2">Décor (greenery, fun cannabis-themed touches like leaf-shaped coasters)</td></tr>
<tr><th colspan="2">Cannabis Essentials</th></tr>
<tr><td>Pre-rolls or joints</td><td>A mix of Sativa, Indica, and hybrid strains</td></tr>
<tr><td>Edibles (gummies, chocolates, or baked goods)</td><td>Vape pens or cartridges</td></tr>
<tr><td>CBD options for those who prefer</td><td>Non-psychoactive effects</td></tr>
<tr><td colspan="2">Smoking accessories (pipes, lighters, rolling papers, grinders)</td></tr>
</table>

Snacks and Drinks	
Sweet options:	
Savory options:	
Non-infused drinks:	
Infused mocktails or teas (optional):	
Activities and Games	
Classic board games (like Jenga or Uno)	Video games (Mario Kart, Jackbox)
Art station (paint, doodle pads, clay)	Music or karaoke setup
After the Party	
What worked well? What could have gone better? How did cannabis enhance the experience?	

Broader Impacts

Effects on Relationships with Pets and Your Community

Cannabis has far-reaching effects that extend beyond the individual, influencing both your relationship with your pets and your connection to your community. As cannabis use becomes increasingly accepted in society, it's important to approach these relationships with awareness, responsibility, and care.

Pets

While cannabis is known to have therapeutic benefits for humans, it's essential to be mindful of how it impacts pets. THC, the psychoactive compound in cannabis, can be toxic to animals, especially dogs and cats. It's crucial to keep all cannabis products out of their reach to avoid accidental ingestion. If you're using cannabis at home, ensure that your pets are safe in a separate area to prevent any accidental exposure. If you suspect that your pet has ingested cannabis, it's important to contact a veterinarian immediately.

However, the non-psychoactive compound CBD can offer health benefits for pets when used responsibly. There are a variety of CBD products on the market designed specifically for animals, aimed at helping with issues like anxiety, pain, and inflammation. These products can help calm pets during stressful situations, such as thunderstorms or trips to the vet, and can even assist with conditions like arthritis or chronic pain. But before introducing any cannabis-based product to your pet's routine, always consult with a veterinarian to ensure it's the right fit for them.

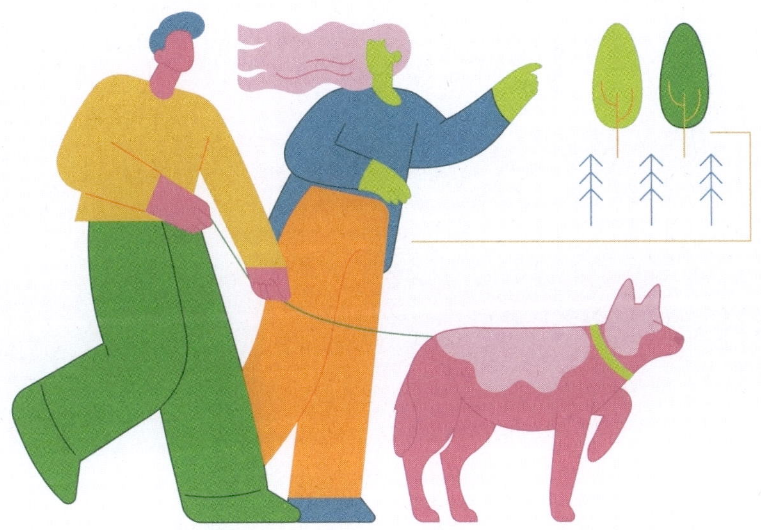

On the other hand, cannabis can also enhance your experience as a pet owner, especially when it comes to creating a deeper bond and being more present in your daily interactions with your pets. The relaxing effects of cannabis can help you slow down, allowing you to appreciate those simple, everyday moments with your furry companions. Whether it's taking a leisurely walk with your dog, feeling more attuned to the world around you, or sinking into a cozy couch cuddle with your cat, cannabis can amplify your sense of connection to your pets. Playtime can also become more fun and engaging when you're in a relaxed state of mind, giving you the space to laugh at your pet's quirky antics and appreciate their personality in a more profound way. For example, after a sesh, we love giving our cat a little catnip and watching him frolic around the room.

Pet CBD Usage Tracker

This tracker helps readers log and monitor their pets' CBD usage, dosage, and outcomes to ensure safe and effective experiences.

How to Use:

1. **Pet's Name:** Record which pet received CBD, especially for multi-pet households.
2. **CBD Product:** Write down the brand, form (oil, treats, etc.), and CBD concentration (e.g., 300mg per bottle).
3. **Dosage:** Track how much you gave (e.g., "1 dropper = 5mg").

4. **Reason for Use:** Examples: anxiety (fireworks, car rides), pain relief (arthritis, surgery), or relaxation.

5. **Effects Noted:** Describe how your pet reacted (e.g., "Calmer during thunderstorm," "Slept better," "No noticeable change").

6. **Next Steps/Adjustments:** Note if you plan to increase or decrease the dosage, switch products, or consult your vet.

Important Note:

Before introducing CBD to your pet, always consult with your veterinarian to ensure it's safe and appropriate for their health needs. Every pet reacts differently to CBD, and factors like weight, age, and existing conditions can influence the right dosage. Your vet can help you choose the best product and approach for your furry friend!

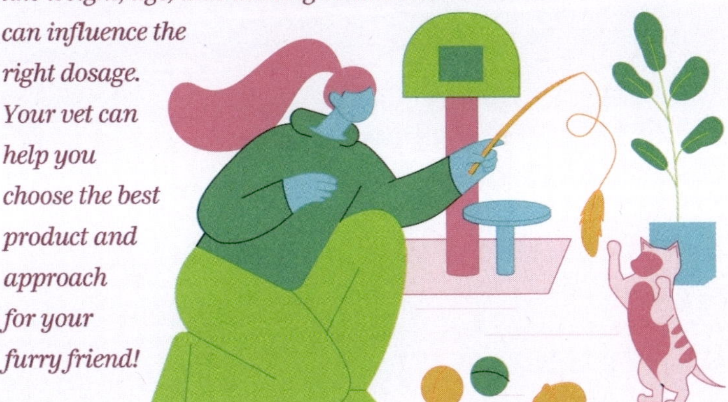

Example Entry:

Date	Pet's Name	CBD Product	Dosage
08/10/2024	Indy	Pawfect CBD Oil (300mg)	1 Dropper

Date	Pet's Name	CBD Product	Dosage

Reason for Use	Effects Noted	Next Steps/Adjustment
Fireworks anxiety	Slept peacefully, no pacing	Continue dose during fireworks

Reason for Use	Effects Noted	Next Steps/Adjustment

Date	Pet's Name	CBD Product	Dosage

Reason for Use	Effects Noted	Next Steps/Adjustment

Community

Cannabis also plays a significant role in shaping relationships with the wider community. As cannabis moves from the fringes to the mainstream, participating in local cannabis events, joining advocacy groups, and supporting responsible consumption can help challenge the stigma that still surrounds its use. By becoming an active member of the cannabis community, whether through volunteering, attending educational events, or simply sharing your personal experiences, you contribute to the normalization of cannabis and help others see it as a natural, beneficial part of life.

The more openly we talk about cannabis, the more we can break down barriers and create an atmosphere of acceptance and understanding. When you share your positive experiences with cannabis–whether it's how it helps you relax, manage stress, or enhance your creativity–you help to foster a supportive, informed environment. This, in turn, helps reduce the negative stereotypes often associated with cannabis users. The more people understand the benefits, the more comfortable they feel using cannabis responsibly and in ways that support their well-being.

Beyond individual experiences, cannabis use can also lead to greater community engagement. Participating in or even hosting cannabis-related events, such as educational sessions, wellness workshops, or local dispensary pop-ups, can bring people together who might otherwise never cross paths. These events offer a space for like-minded individuals to share knowledge, stories, and support for responsible cannabis consumption. They also serve as powerful platforms to advocate for the continued legalization and normalization of cannabis, ensuring that future generations benefit from an open and inclusive cannabis culture.

By thoughtfully incorporating cannabis into your relationship with your community, you can play a part in shaping a more understanding, inclusive world. Cannabis can be a tool for building stronger connections, both with the people closest to you and with those who share similar values and interests.

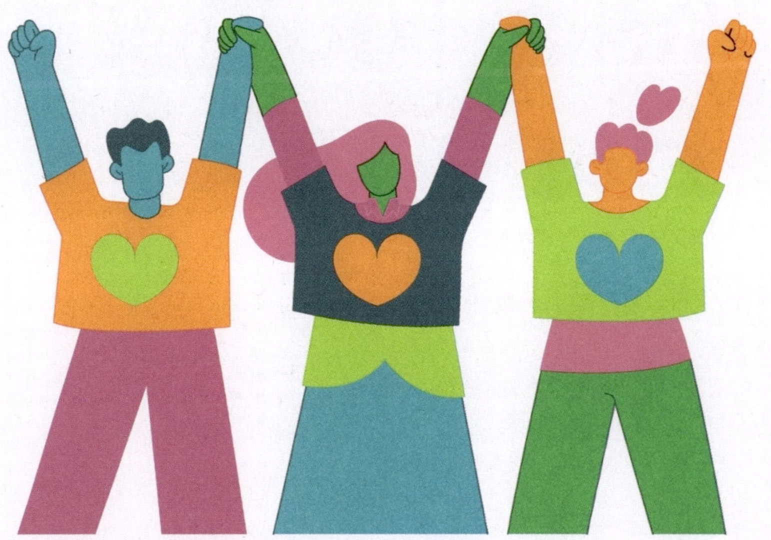

Conclusion

Cannabis as a Tool for Happiness, Wellness, Connection

As we conclude this journey through the many facets of cannabis, it's clear that this plant offers more than a recreational experience. Cannabis has the potential to enhance relationships, improve personal well-being, and unlock creative potential when used intentionally. Its role in the wellness world is just beginning to be fully understood, and it's up to each of us to explore how it can fit into our lives in meaningful, positive ways.

Enhancing Relationships

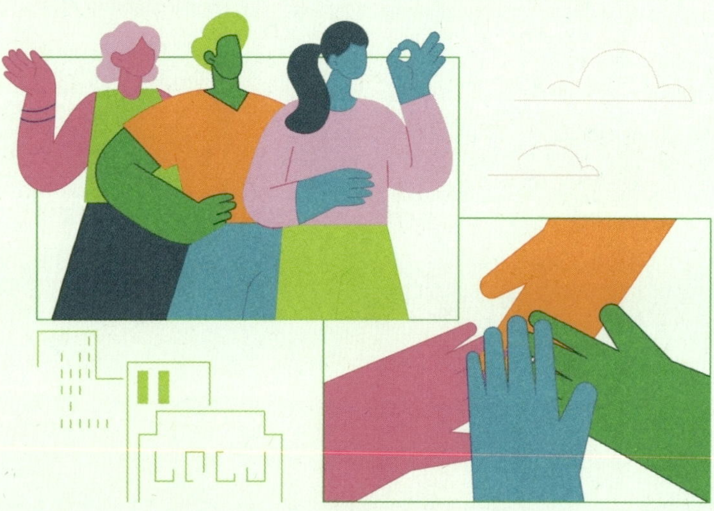

When it comes to human connection, cannabis offers a unique ability to bring people together. Whether you're sharing a joint with friends, deepening intimacy with a partner, or finding common ground with family members across generations, cannabis can create an environment for honest, open communication. The plant's relaxing effects can dissolve barriers, promote vulnerability, and foster shared experiences. Research supports this as well–studies show that cannabis use can enhance emotional bonding, helping individuals connect with their partners and friends on a deeper level, and fostering feelings of empathy and emotional openness.

Throughout this journey, we've seen how cannabis can play a key role in breaking down social walls and facilitating deeper, more meaningful conversations. But it's not just about enhancing interpersonal interactions–it's also about building a better relationship with yourself. Mindfully incorporating cannabis into your routine allows you to reconnect with your body and mind, find moments of stillness, and nurture your well-being. Whether you use it to unwind after a stressful day, spark creativity, or simply help you feel more present, cannabis can be a tool to support your emotional health and mental clarity.

Personal Well-Being and Self-Discovery

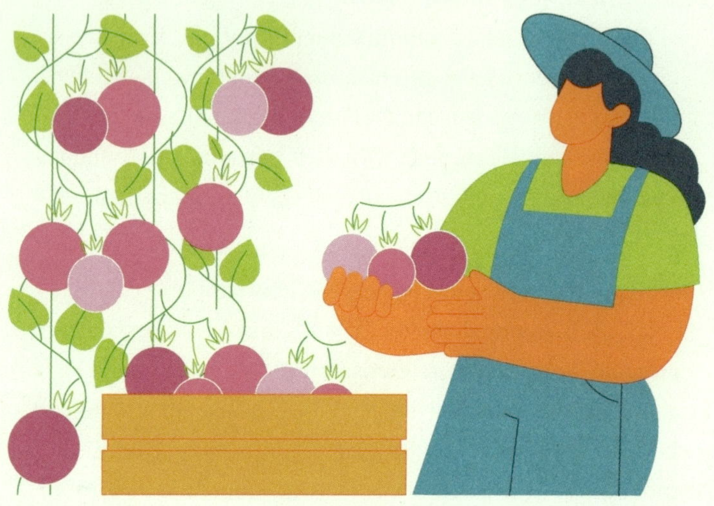

Cannabis has long been used for its therapeutic benefits, and there's growing evidence to support its role in promoting well-being. Scientific research shows that cannabis, particularly CBD, can help reduce anxiety, alleviate chronic pain, and improve sleep. THC, the psychoactive compound in cannabis, has been shown to increase dopamine levels, contributing to feelings of happiness and relaxation. But it's important to remember that cannabis isn't a cure-all. It's a tool that, when used responsibly, can complement other wellness practices such as mindfulness, physical activity, yoga, and healthy eating. Integrating cannabis into a holistic self-care routine enhances its potential to support your overall well-being.

While cannabis can offer immediate relief, it also promotes long-term benefits when used thoughtfully. Many people find that using cannabis to support their mental health and emotional state can help them achieve a greater sense of balance. However, just as with any wellness tool, moderation is key. It's crucial to stay informed about how cannabis affects you and recognize when its use may become excessive or lead to negative outcomes, like anxiety or dependence.

Creativity and Mindfulness

Cannabis is also a powerful catalyst for creativity. Many artists, writers, musicians, and thinkers have turned to cannabis for inspiration, with anecdotal evidence suggesting that it unlocks new ways of thinking and helps individuals approach problems with a fresh perspective. THC has been shown to enhance divergent thinking, which is the ability to generate creative ideas by exploring many possible solutions. For those in creative fields, cannabis can break through mental blocks and open the door to new creative insights.

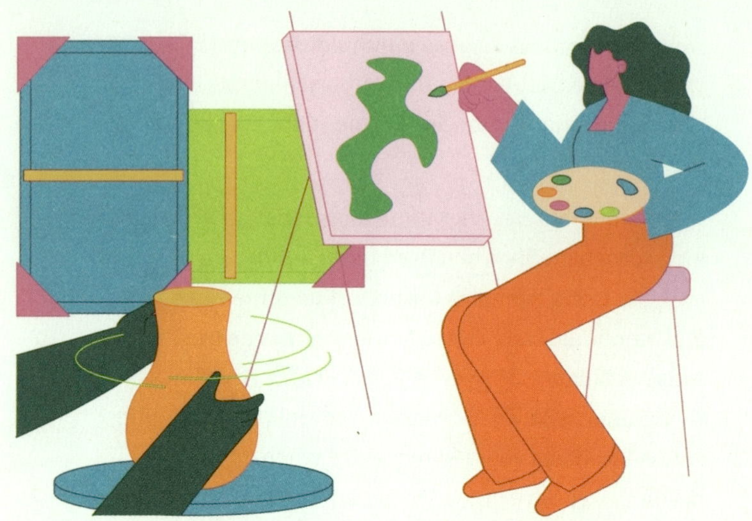

But cannabis isn't just for the artist—it can be a tool for anyone looking to engage their mind differently. Whether it's brainstorming, finding new ways to solve problems at work, or simply exploring new hobbies, cannabis can foster mental openness and encourage new approaches. It offers a chance to step outside the usual patterns of thought and approach challenges with a more fluid and innovative mindset.

Potential Risks and Responsible Use

While cannabis has many benefits, it's essential to approach it with care and mindfulness. Like any substance, it comes with potential risks, especially if used irresponsibly or excessively. Overuse can lead to dependency, and for some individuals, especially those with a history of mental health issues such as anxiety or depression, cannabis can exacerbate symptoms, leading to feelings of paranoia or heightened anxiety.

To use cannabis responsibly, it's important to recognize your limits and listen to your body. Start with small doses, especially if you're new to cannabis, and pay attention to how it affects you. If you notice any negative side effects, it's important to adjust your usage accordingly or consult with a healthcare professional. Understanding how cannabis impacts your body and mind is key to ensuring that it remains a positive, enriching experience rather than a source of stress or discomfort.

A New Perspective on Cannabis

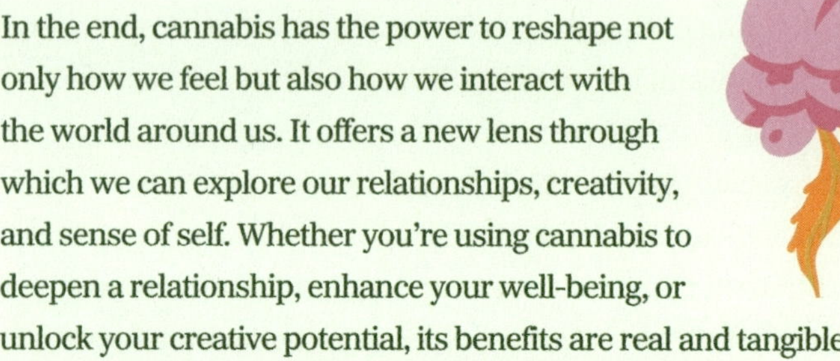

In the end, cannabis has the power to reshape not only how we feel but also how we interact with the world around us. It offers a new lens through which we can explore our relationships, creativity, and sense of self. Whether you're using cannabis to deepen a relationship, enhance your well-being, or unlock your creative potential, its benefits are real and tangible.

As societal acceptance of cannabis continues to grow, so too does the opportunity to use this powerful plant for personal growth, joy, and connection. By embracing cannabis with intention, we can discover new perspectives on life and enrich our journey individually and collectively.

So, as you continue your exploration of cannabis, remember to stay curious, stay open, and let this plant guide you toward a richer, more connected, and fulfilling life.

Explore, enjoy, and let cannabis be a positive, transformative part of your wellness journey.

As you close this book, we hope you're walking away with new ideas, deeper connections, and a fresh perspective on what cannabis can bring to your life. The art of the high life is a journey—one that's personal, ever-evolving, and full of opportunities for growth, joy, and connection.

To help you celebrate your progress and keep exploring, we've included this **Gratitude Journal** to reflect on your experiences and set intentions for the future. Take a moment to honor how far you've come and look forward to what's next on your cannabis journey.

Gratitude Journal
Reflecting on Your Cannabis Journey

Reflection Prompts

1. **What's your favorite cannabis memory?**

   Describe a sesh, moment, or experience where cannabis brought you joy, connection, or peace.

   ____

   ____

   ____

   ____

   ____

2. **How has cannabis improved your daily life?**

Think about areas like your mood, sleep, creativity, relationships, or overall well-being.

3. **What's a challenge cannabis has helped you overcome?**

Did it help with stress, anxiety, pain management, or finding time for yourself? Reflect on the growth you've experienced.

4. **What are you most grateful for in your cannabis journey so far?**

   Has it brought you closer to others, inspired you creatively, or made life's simple moments feel more meaningful?

5. **What goals do you want to achieve with cannabis in the future?**

   Examples: Mindful consumption, exploring new products, hosting a sesh with friends, or incorporating it into your wellness routines.

6. **What are three ways you can use cannabis with more intention moving forward?**

Example: "Keep a journal of my experiences."

Example: "Try cannabis before meditation for deeper focus."

Example: "Incorporate it into date nights for a more relaxed, bonding experience."

Sketch how cannabis makes you *feel!*

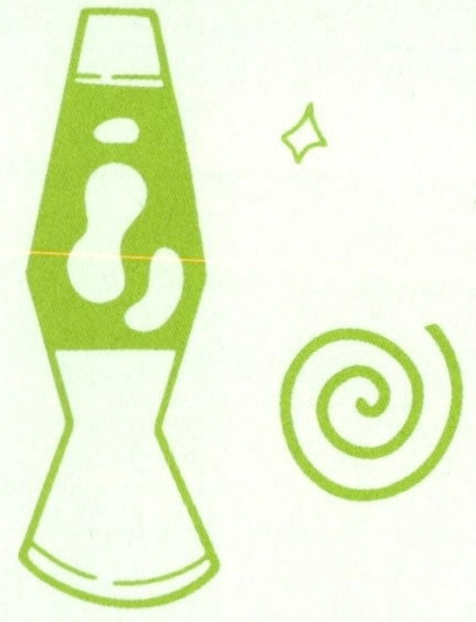

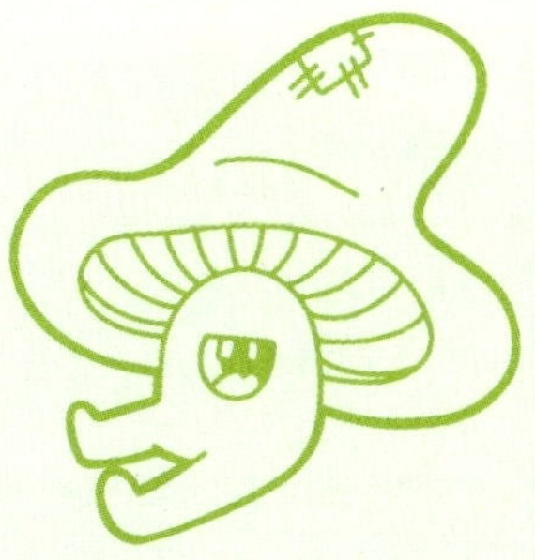

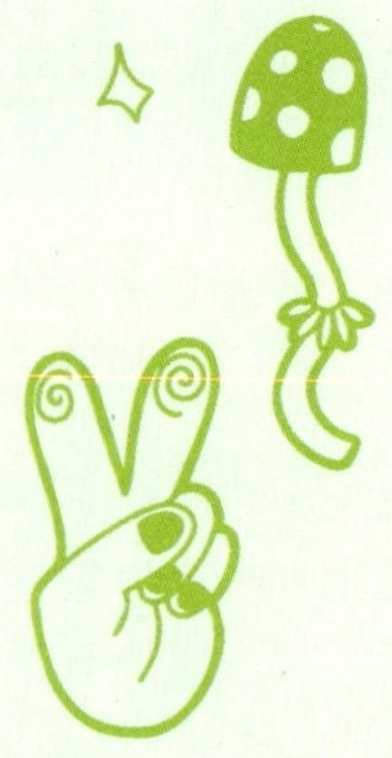

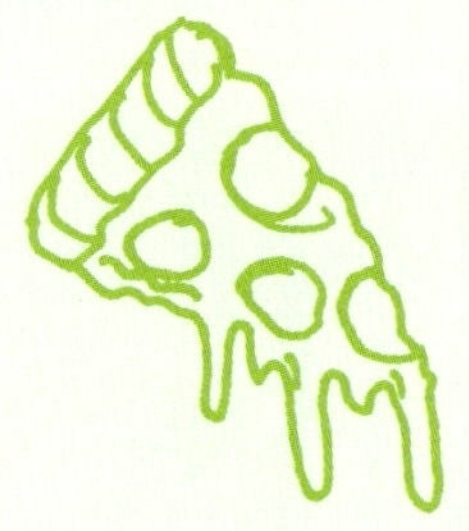

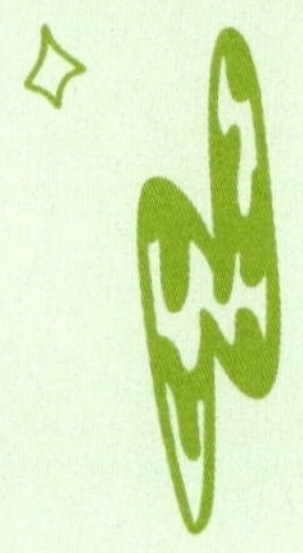

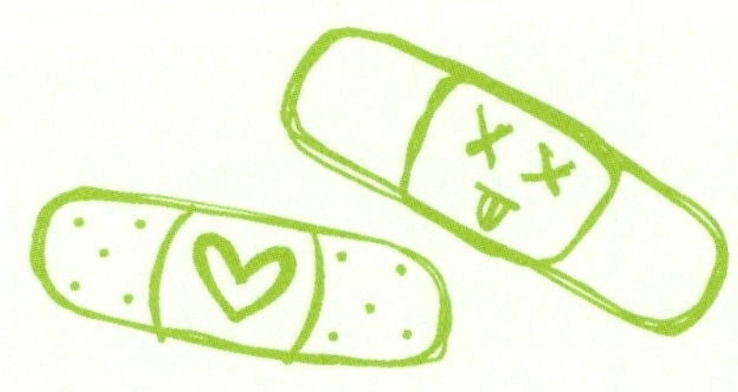

Appendices

Safe Consumption Practices

Ensuring safe and enjoyable cannabis consumption is essential for a positive experience. Here's a quick guide for some key practices to keep in mind:

1. **Start Low and Go Slow:** Begin with a small dose, especially if you're new to a particular form of cannabis. Edibles and concentrates can be particularly potent, so it's wise to start with a lower dose and wait to gauge the effects before consuming more.

2. **Know Your Source:** Ensure that your cannabis comes from a reputable source. Quality and consistency can vary, so buying from licensed dispensaries or trusted suppliers helps ensure you're getting a safe product.

3. **Understand the Delivery Method:** Different methods of consumption have different onset times and durations. Smoking and vaping typically have faster onset times, while edibles and tinctures can take longer to take effect. Adjust your consumption method based on your needs and preferences.

4. **Stay Hydrated:** Cannabis can cause dry mouth, so keep water handy to stay hydrated. This is particularly important if you're consuming cannabis in a social setting or engaging in physical activity.

5. **Avoid Mixing with Alcohol or Other Substances:** Combining cannabis with alcohol or other substances can alter its effects and potentially increase risks. If you're new to cannabis, it's best to avoid mixing until you understand how it affects you on its own.

6. **Secure Your Products:** Keep cannabis products out of reach of children and pets. Store them in a safe, discreet place to prevent accidental consumption and ensure safety.

7. **Be Mindful of Your Environment:** Consume cannabis in a safe, comfortable setting where you feel at ease. Avoid operating vehicles or heavy machinery under the influence to ensure safety.

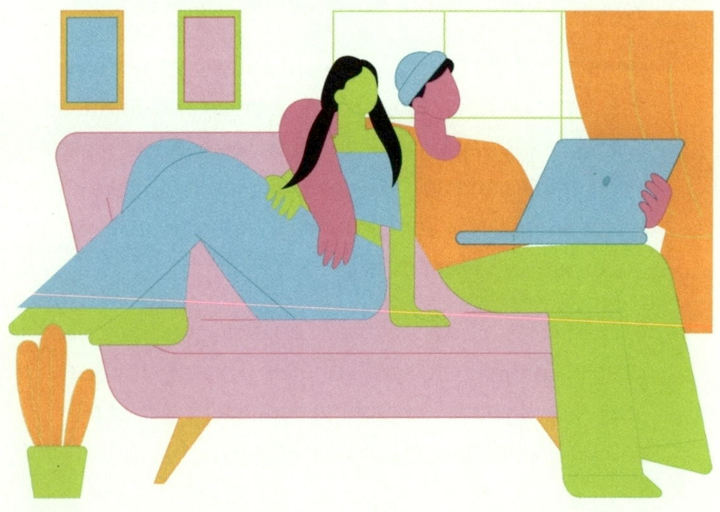

Legal Considerations by Region

Cannabis laws vary widely depending on your location. Here's a general guide to understanding where and how you can legally consume cannabis:

1. United States

In the US, recreational cannabis use is legal in twenty-three states, typically for adults aged twenty-one and older. However, public consumption remains mostly prohibited, with some states beginning to open consumption lounges where cannabis use is allowed. Medicinal cannabis is legal in thirty-eight states, but each state has a set of qualifying conditions and regulations, often requiring a medical card for access. It's important to note that federal law prohibits crossing state lines with cannabis, even between states where it is legal.

2. Canada

In Canada, recreational cannabis has been fully legal nationwide since 2018, with the legal age for use set at either eighteen or nineteen, depending on the province. Consumers are allowed to possess up to thirty grams of cannabis in public, and provincial regulations determine where cannabis can be purchased and consumed. Medicinal cannabis has been legal for years and is available with a prescription from licensed producers. Public consumption rules vary, with some provinces permitting use in places where tobacco is allowed while others restrict it to private property.

3. Europe

In Europe, cannabis laws vary significantly by country. In the Netherlands, cannabis is decriminalized for personal use, and coffee shops in cities like Amsterdam legally sell cannabis for on-site consumption. In Spain, private cannabis clubs are legal, but public consumption and sales remain illegal. Germany is in the process of legalizing recreational cannabis use under strict guidelines. In the United Kingdom, cannabis remains illegal for recreational purposes but is available medicinally with a prescription.

4. Australia

In Australia, recreational cannabis use is only legal in the Australian Capital Territory (ACT), where individuals can possess and cultivate small amounts for personal use, though sale remains illegal. Medicinal cannabis is legal nationwide, but access is typically through a government-approved prescription program. Public consumption is prohibited, and the use of cannabis is restricted to private residences, with significant penalties for violating these rules.

5. Other International Locations

Cannabis laws are diverse and can change rapidly. If you're planning to travel internationally, it's crucial to stay informed about the local regulations. In some countries, even small amounts of cannabis can lead to severe penalties, including hefty fines or imprisonment. While some destinations may be more lenient or even allow medical use, others have zero-tolerance policies. Research the current legal status of cannabis in your destination before you go, and remember that what's legal at home might be strictly prohibited abroad.

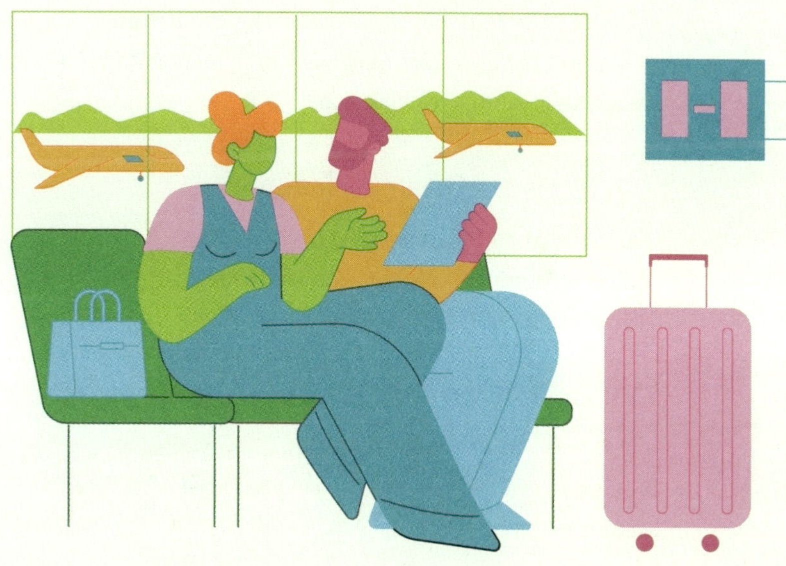

Recommended Resources

For those interested in further exploring the world of cannabis, the following resources offer valuable information:

Websites

- **Leafly:** Provides strain reviews, industry news, and educational resources on cannabis.
- **Weedmaps:** Offers information on dispensaries, strains, and cannabis-related services.
- **NORML:** The National Organization for the Reform of Marijuana Laws offers advocacy information and updates on cannabis legislation.

Communities

- **YouTube and Instagram:** Join our That High Couple online community for cannabis culture and education.
- **Reddit's r/trees:** A community for cannabis enthusiasts to share experiences and advice.
- **Local Meetups:** Look for local cannabis events or meetups to connect with others in your area who share an interest in cannabis.

Acknowledgments

To our incredible community: thank you for being the heart and soul of this journey. Every like, comment, share, and message has fueled our passion and pushed us to create something meaningful. This book wouldn't exist without your support and enthusiasm. To you all, and the team at Mango Publishing, thank you for being a part of our story and for making everything we do so rewarding. Here's to all the good vibes to come.

With love,

Alice & Clark

About the Authors

Alice and Clark Campbell, better known as That High Couple, are the dynamic duo behind a thriving community dedicated to cannabis education and normalization. Together, they've built a space where seasoned enthusiasts and curious newcomers alike can explore the world of cannabis with humor, insight, and authenticity.

Through their content, Alice and Clark aim to shatter stereotypes and highlight the many ways cannabis can enrich lives–whether it's by deepening relationships, sparking creativity, or fostering self-care. Based in Seattle, they continue to document their journey with their two cats, Bramble and Biscuit, and their ever-growing collection of glass bongs and houseplants. *The Art of the High Life* is their first book, a labor of love inspired by their mission to spread knowledge and reduce the stigma around this incredible plant.

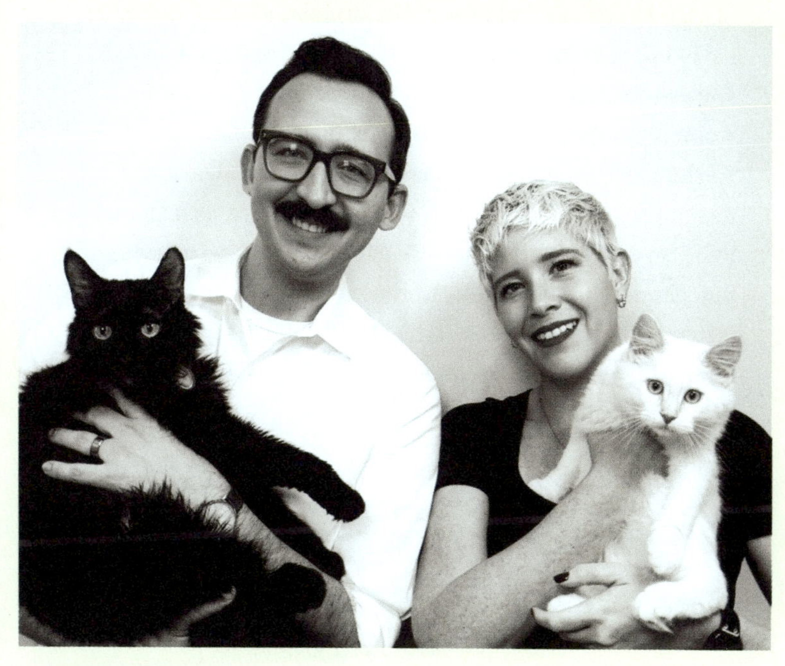

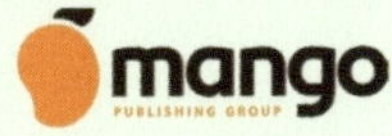

Mango Publishing, established in 2014, publishes an eclectic list of books by diverse authors—both new and established voices—on topics ranging from business, personal growth, women's empowerment, LGBTQ+ studies, health, and spirituality to history, popular culture, time management, decluttering, lifestyle, mental wellness, aging, and sustainable living. We were named 2019 *and* 2020's #1 fastest growing independent publisher by *Publishers Weekly*. Our success is driven by our main goal, which is to publish high-quality books that will entertain readers as well as make a positive difference in their lives.

Our readers are our most important resource; we value your input, suggestions, and ideas. We'd love to hear from you—after all, we are publishing books for you!

Please stay in touch with us and follow us at:

Facebook: Mango Publishing
Twitter: @MangoPublishing
Instagram: @MangoPublishing
LinkedIn: Mango Publishing
Pinterest: Mango Publishing
Newsletter: mangopublishinggroup.com/newsletter

Join us on Mango's journey to reinvent publishing, one book at a time.